Gastric Band Hypnosis for Women

How to Burn Calories Fast and Lose Weight with Powerful Self-Hypnosis Techniques. Lose Weight Effectively with Professional Guided Hypnosis Sessions

Elizabeth Collins

Table of Contents

Introduction

Hypnosis is rewiring your brain to add or to change your daily routine starting from your basic instincts. This happens due to the fact that while you are in a hypnotic state you are more susceptible to suggestions by the person who put you in this state. In the case of self-hypnosis, the person who made you enter the trance of hypnotism is yourself. Thus, the only person who can give you suggestions that can change your attitude in this method is you and you alone.

Again, you must forget the misconception that hypnosis is like sleeping because if it is then it would be impossible to give autosuggestions to yourself. Try to think about it like being in a very vivid daydream where you are capable of controlling every aspect of the situation you are in. This gives you the ability to change anything that may bother and hinder you to achieve the best possible result. If you are able to pull it off properly, then the possibility of improving yourself after a constant practice of the method will just be a few steps away.

Career

People say that motivation is the key to improve in your career. But no matter how you love your career, you must admit that there are aspects in your work that you really do not like doing. Even if it is a fact that you are good in the other tasks, there is that one duty that you dread. And every time you encounter this specific chore you seem to be slowed down and thus lessening your productivity at work. This is where self-hypnosis comes into play.

The first thing you need to do is find that task you do not like. In some cases there might be multiple of them depending on your personality and how you feel about your job. Now, try to look at why you do not like that task and do simple research on how to make the job a lot simpler. You can then start conditioning yourself to use the simple method every time you do the job.

After you are able to condition your state of mind to do the task, each time you encounter it will become the trigger for your trance and thus giving you the ability to perform it better. You will not be able to tell the difference since you will not mind it at all. Your coworkers and superiors though will definitely notice the change in your work style and in your productivity.

Family

It is easy to improve in a career. But to improve your relationship with your family can be a little tricky. Yet, self-hypnosis can still reprogram you to interact with your family members better by modifying how you react to the way they act. You will have the ability to adjust your way of thinking depending on the situation. This then allows you to respond in the most positive way possible, no matter how dreadful the scenario may be.

If you are in a fight with your husband/wife, for example, the normal reaction is to flare up and face fire with fire. The problem with this approach is it usually engulfs the entire relationship which might eventually lead up to separation. Being in a hypnotic state in this instance can help you think clearly and change the impulse of saying the words without thinking through. Anger will still be there, of course, that is the healthy way. But anger now under self-hypnosis can be channeled and stop being a raging inferno, you can turn it into a steady bonfire that can help you and your partner find common ground for whatever issue you are facing. The same applies in dealing with a sibling or children. If you are able to condition your mind to think more rationally or to get into the perspective of others, then you can have better family/friends' relationships.

Health and Physical Activities

Losing weight can be the most common reason why people will use self-hypnosis in terms of health and physical activities. But this is just one part of it. Self-hypnosis can give you a lot more to improve this aspect of your life. It works the same way while working out.

Most people tend to give up their exercise program due to the exhaustion they think they can no longer take. But through self-hypnosis, you will be able to tell yourself that the exhaustion is lessened and thus allowing you to finish the entire routine. Keep in mind though that your mind must never be conditioned to forget exhaustion, it must only not mind it until the end of the exercise. Forgetting it completely might lead you to not stopping to work out until your energy is depleted. It becomes counterproductive in this case.

Having a healthy diet can also be influenced by self-hypnosis. Conditioning your mind to avoid unhealthy food can be done. Thus, hypnosis will be triggered each you are tempted to eat a meal you are conditioned to consider as unhealthy. Your eating habit then can change to benefit you to improve your overall health.

Mental, Emotional and Spiritual Needs

Since self-hypnosis deals directly in how you think, it is then no secret that it can greatly improve your mental, emotional and spiritual needs. A clear mind can give your brain the ability to have more rational thoughts. Rationality then leads to better decision making and easy absorption and retention of information you might need to improve your mental capacity. You must set your expectations, though; this does not work like magic that can turn you into a genius. The process takes time depending on how far you want to go, how much you want to achieve. Thus, the effects will only be limited by how much you are able to condition your mind.

In terms of emotional needs, self-hypnosis cannot make you feel differently in certain situations. But it can condition you to take in each scenario a little lighter and make you deal with them better. Others think that getting rid of emotion can be the best course of action if you are truly able to rewire your brain. But they seem to forget that even though rational thinking is often influenced negatively by emotion, it is still necessary for you to decide on things basing on the common ethics and aesthetics of the real world. Self-hypnosis then can channel your emotion to work in a more positive way in terms of decision making and dealing with emotional hurdles and problems.

Spiritual need on the other hand is far easier to influence when it comes to doing self-hypnosis. As a matter of fact, most people with spiritual beliefs are able to do self-hypnosis each time they practice what they believe in. A deep prayer, for instance, is a way to self-hypnotize yourself to enter the trance to feel closer to a Divine existence. Chanting and meditation done by other religions also leads and have the same goal. Even the songs during a mass or praise and worship triggers self-hypnosis depending if the person allows them to do so.

Still, the improvements can only be achieved if you condition yourself that you are ready to accept them. The willingness to put an effort must also be there. An effortless hypnosis will only create the illusion that you are improving and thus will not give you the satisfaction of achieving your goal in reality.

How hypnosis can help resolve childhood issues

Another issue that hypnosis can help you with are problems from our past. If you have had traumatic situations from your childhood days, then you may have issues in all areas of your adult life. Unresolved issues from your past can lead to anxiety and depression in your later years. Childhood trauma is dangerous because it can alter many things in the brain both psychologically and chemically.

The most vital thing to remember about trauma from your childhood is that given a harmless and caring environment in which the child's vital needs for physical safety, importance, emotional security and attention are met, the damage that trauma and abuse cause can be eased and relieved. Safe and dependable relationships are also a dynamic component in healing the effects of childhood trauma in adulthood and make an atmosphere in which the brain can safely start the process of recovery.

Pure Hypnoanalysis is the lone most effective method of treatment available in the world today, for the resolution of phobias, anxiety, depression, fears, psychological and emotional problems/symptoms and eating disorders. It is a highly advanced form of hypnoanalysis (referred to as analytical hypnotherapy or hypno-analysis). Hypnoanalysis, in its numerous forms, is practiced all over the world; this method of hypnotherapy can completely resolve the foundation of anxieties in the unconscious mind, leaving the individual free of their symptoms for life.

There is a deeper realism active at all times around us and inside us. This reality commands that we must come to this world to find happiness, and every so often that our inner child stands in our way. This is by no means intentional; however, it desires to reconcile wounds from the past or address damaging philosophies which were troubling to us as children.

So disengaging the issues that upset us from earlier in our lives we have to find a way to bond with our internal child, we then need to assist in rebuilding this part of us which will, in turn, help us to be rid of all that has been hindering us from moving on.

Connecting with your inner child may seem like something

that may be hard or impossible to do, especially since they may be a part that has long been buried. It is a fairly easy exercise to do and can even be done right now. You will need about 20 minutes to complete this exercise. Here's what you do: find a quiet spot where you won't be disturbed and find pictures of you as a child if you think it may help.

Breathe in and loosen your clothing if you have to. Inhale deeply into your abdomen and exhale, repeat until you feel yourself getting relaxed; you may close your eyes and focus on getting less tense. Feel your forehead and head relax, let your face become relaxed and relax your shoulders. Allow your body to be limp and loose while you breathe slowly. Keep breathing slowly as you let all of your tension float away.

Now slowly count from 10 to 0 in your mind and try to think of a place from your childhood. The image doesn't have to be crystal clear right now but try to focus on exactly how you remember it and keep that image in mind. Imagine yourself as a child and imagine observing younger you; think about your clothes, expression, hair, etc. In your mind go and meet yourself, introduce yourself to you.

Chapter 1: Building the Foundation

It is important to gain insight into the internal and external influences that form you're eating habits, and to cultivate intrinsic motivation partly by interacting with your values. But modifying your behavior will remain discouragingly difficult—not because you are necessarily lazy or self-destructive, but because eating is an ingrained habit that you've been doing for decades.

Researchers have been zeroing in on the neuroscience in recent years, which develops patterns and keeps them in place. Doing an action in a certain way, over time, slowly develops neural pathways within the brain and the behavior is automatic, something we do without thought. This method, known as procedural learning, occurs for routine tasks that most of us learn as children, including brushing our teeth and tying our shoes, and it can occur for eating habits that we've come to follow almost instinctively, whether they're healthy or unhealthy. It is easier to think about any learned behavior as a bundled answer that gets wired into our brains. Some packaged responses include brain parts called reward centers, which make them even more tenacious and complex.

Smoking, gambling, drug intake, and consuming high-sugar or high-fat foods fall under this group.

Let us look at a popular one that most of us can recall learning to understand how bundled responses work: driving. If you learned as a teenager, you probably still remember those herky-jerky first attempts that took all your concentration and energy, along with the look of thinly veiled fear on your mother's face, dad, older sibling or driving instructor sitting in the passenger seat. But over time, the different specialized skills needed to drive, steering, accelerating, or braking, changing gears, slowly fused into a smooth, coherent whole. Driving has become automatic, something you do without worrying a great deal about. It is now a packed response after years of practice.

Like driving, eating habits can, over time, be stored as packed responses in our brains. From a health viewpoint, it is worth changing habits to open a Coke every night when you get home or pop chips into your mouth when finishing work tasks. But on a physiological level, eating habits like those are what the brain and body know how to do.

Packaged eating reactions are more complex than driving or tying your shoes, containing far more chemicals in the body— peptides, hormones, and neurotransmitters. Maybe more important, whatever connections you have developed between eating and emotions can also be packed together: for example, reaching for carbohydrates when you are upset is a popular packed answer. Sometimes, these bundled responses are programmed, incorporated, and stored in our brain physiology. Such connections have probably in the past helped you cope in some way. However, if done too much, the costs outweigh the benefits, and it might be time to develop new relationships.

Rewiring the Brain

The good news is our brains are "soft-wired," not hard-wired. They have neuroplasticity with new neural pathways, which means they can be rewired. That is not a quick or simple process—it takes time, intent and practice. To undo a packaged response such as eating and its associations, you need a method to isolate the package first and foremost.

Enter consciousness. A theory based on everyday practice, consciousness cultivates the mindset and skills required to pick out the individual pieces of a compressed response such as eating—and the resources to improve it.

The skills you will learn here are a type of applied conscientiousness that blends ancient tradition with modern science. The nature of practice—meditation of mindfulness—originates from the teachings of Buddhism. In the 1970s, Jon

Kabat-Zinn, Ph.D., developed a program at the University of Massachusetts Medical Center that translated some of those teachings into a secular context, Mindfulness-Based Stress Reduction (MBSR). MBSR has been developed to help people manage stress, pain, and several acute and chronic diseases. MBSR's remarkable popularity it is now being taught at more than 200 health centers and its effects have been confirmed in several studies, has given rise to similar types of applied knowledge, like the mindful eating system you are using.

The heart of the practice of mindfulness is to pay attention consciously, with empathy and curiosity to what you are doing in the present—in both your body and mind. It may not sound like a big deal, but paying attention is the opposite of what we are conditioned to do (to stay unconscious) by both our social culture and our practiced prepared reactions, and the opposite of what most of us do. Practicing mindfulness can disrupt unconscious and reactive behavior—which involves unhealthy eating for many people. You begin to realize the subtle underlying feelings, emotions, and physical sensations that drive the behaviors by practicing mindfulness, and that knowledge is the beginning of improvement.

When you pick apart a packaged answer related to food, you know there are certain facets of automatic actions that you have power over. You discover that what seems like a single event—for example, overeating at lunch—is, in fact, a collection of tiny "micro-events," all connected. You might still be bombarded on your way to your office by the seductive scent of freshly baked muffins at the bakery, but you can pause before you walk in, buy one, and wolf it down; in that pause, you remember and feel the power to make another choice. And paying attention can be creative, easy as it sounds.

However, paying attention is not automatic. It acts, in the form of daily meditation and practice.

Taking the Package Apart: Sensations, Thoughts, and Emotions

Undoing the bundled answers that do not serve you well starts by tuning in to what's going on in your body and mind—specifically, physical stimuli, feelings and emotions.

We're always "in our heads" rather than our bodies, so it provides some valuable knowledge to tun into our bodies. For example, experiencing hunger and fullness signals from your body and the way food tastes will dramatically alter you're eating experience. Or you might find that in the afternoons, after sitting all day at your office, you feel a wave of exhaustion and your shoulders start to ache—and that you prefer to respond by going to the vending machine and buying M&Ms. Noticing stimuli as they arise helps you to respond in a healthier manner, which can avoid the domino effect that contributes to unhealthy eating. For example, if you feel the afternoon tiredness and pain, you can respond by taking a 10-minute walk outside, instead of eating M&Ms.

Identifying your thoughts that sound easy, but for many people it's challenging because we prefer to connect with our thoughts instead of identifying them for what they are: separate mental "events" containing information— information that may or may not be valid and may or may not be helpful. Beliefs—ideas so deeply rooted that we consider them to be real—are especially tenacious. Suppose you are eating a piece of cheesecake, and only "think" that you've done it because you don't have self-control. That so-called information is conviction, not reality. It is important to know that our thoughts can lead us astray. When we think we should be that way, or need other stuff, we sometimes convey patterns or messages absorbed from others or our culture in general. Such convictions are not only always unfounded, they do not serve us well, either. You may ask when you accept a thought or opinion, do I know that to be true? How does the thought make me feel? How do I act on that idea? Take a woman in the dressing room, for example, who actually "knows" that she should be a size 6. Whence comes this "knowledge?" What is it that makes her have the belief?

How is she acting upon that belief?

You should practice observing your thoughts during meditation. You will be able to note your emotions in your daily life when you get good at that. And that gives you the chance to analyze them, challenge their validity and alter the actions that motivate those thoughts. In the conventional practice of mindfulness, people learn to observe thoughts as they form—and then the thoughts fade away without requiring a response. If you know in applied awareness whether a thought is false or unhelpful, you can only watch the thought disappear (as in conventional awareness)—or you can alter the thought if it makes you improve your behavior. Suppose your office, for example, is stacked high with paperwork. "My office is something of a mess. I'll never be able to clean it up, "you think—and you'll go to get a snack in response to that thought (even though you're not hungry). When you understand this pattern, you may consciously analyze your thoughts and alter them. The self-defeating thinking, "I'm never going to be able to clean it up," may turn into "I'm going to waste ten minutes sorting the papers on my desk." As for feelings, we are all feeling them but don't really know how to define them or what to do about them. That is partly cultural. Compared to other cultures, our emphasis is very much on problem-solving and doing (instead of being) and thinking rather than feeling. We do not know what feelings can do. So, when feelings are met, they're usually just optimistic ones. The negative ones are messy, uncomfortable, and unreasonable and most of us are learning very little knowledge or skills on how to handle them on our journey to adulthood. Some emotions tend to be shied away from, devalued, and even punished from an early age, such as sadness and rage. Children are told explicitly and implicitly, in certain families and at school, to "be good," not to scream, not to be angry, and not to be afraid.

Under certain conditions, the repression of emotions will mean that they explode in others. We are overcome by the flip side of rejecting feelings, which is also normal. Often people get caught in frustration, snapping at their spouses and kids; or in panic, imagining the most severe cause of unexplained physical symptoms possible. We over-identify with emotions as with thoughts and can't see them for what they are for. Many people respond to emotions—whether they're overwhelming or suppressed.

Mindfulness provides a middle way to deal with feelings, between the extremes of being ignored and swept away by them. As with emotions, the feelings can be felt when holding a wedge of distance—we call this being the Observer. You can see feelings for what they are—and benefit from them when you do so.

You will help improve your eating habits in a variety of ways by being mindful of your inner world—sensations, feelings, and emotions—through mindfulness.

Chapter 2: Overcoming Trauma, Anxiety, and Depression Meditation

Trauma, anxiety, and depression are all difficult things to have to deal with. If you experience one or more of these mental illnesses, then you know that it can be a struggle to get a restful night's sleep.

Anxious thoughts of your past or worries over what might happen tomorrow can really make it hard for you to stay relaxed all throughout the night. Even when you are sleeping, you might have constant nightmares that make it hard for you to feel comfortable in your own bed. In this meditation, we are going to take you through trauma. We are going to make it easier for you to be able to understand how to heal from some of these processes.

What you should know before getting into the meditation is that this is not going to be an instant cure. Mental illness does not go away with the snap of your fingers. It is a constant struggle to find the right mindset to overcome some of your biggest issues. This is a beginner exercise that is going to help unlock some parts of your brain needed to heal. There is a trigger warning for this meditation. We will be talking about wounds and trauma. If at any time your mind seems to wander somewhere dark and you do not understand how to pull yourself from this, feel free to stop and move and do something that distracts you.

Of course, the point of this meditation is going to make sure that you are calm and at peace, but we cannot always help where our minds wander sometimes. If you get stuck in a panic, then remember to simply participate in more breathing exercises.

This meditation will help you heal and find the peace that you need to move on from some of your most challenging issues.

Make sure you are in a comfortable place because towards the end, we are going to encourage you to fall asleep. Keep an open mind and allow your thoughts to flow freely.

Meditation for Quieting Trauma, Depression, and Anxiety

After you have a physical wound on your body, there are four stages of healing that occur. These stages help to ensure that the wound does not get any worse and that it heals properly so that the rest of your body can still function. When we experience something traumatic or endure consistent depression and anxiety, it can be like a wound on your soul. These mental wounds do not have big ugly scars, like a scrape on your knee or cut on your face might. We must remember, however, that these scars are still there.

These mental wounds are something that we still need to treat properly. In this meditation, we are going to help you understand how you can self-heal so that you can finally get the peace you need at night. Too often we lie awake thinking of the terrible things that we've experienced. How frequently do you find it almost impossible to actually get a restful night's sleep without waking up several times, playing a certain traumatic experience over and over again in your mind? You don't have to be a prisoner of your own experiences anymore. It is time to learn how you can best heal so that these wounds don't hurt.

Begin focusing on your breath right now. This is a great meditation to do before bed, but anytime that you need to be more relaxed, after dealing with trauma, anxiety, or depression is perfectly fine as well. Ensure that there are no distractions around you. You don't want any people, pets, music, sounds, sights, or anything else to keep you from being able to drift into a healthy and deep sleep. Feel as the air comes in and out of your body. Already, you can notice the way in which your body does what it can to ensure that you're getting taken care of properly. Even without us thinking about it, our bodies are constantly giving us the right things needed to survive.

We breathe, we digest, we live, we pump blood, and our heart beats. All of this continues to happen without us even having to think about it.

We do some of the work, but our body really comes in and does the rest. It knows exactly how to heal itself as well.

Think about this as you continue to breathe in and out. Breathe in through your nose and out through your mouth. This is a great way to keep you focused on your body. This is the method that you can use to ensure that you aren't thinking too hard about all that is negative for you.

Breathe in again, and out again. Breathe in through your nose for five, four, three, two, and one. Breathe out through your mouth for one, two, three, four, and five. Continue to breathe like this throughout the entire meditation.

When you get a cut or a scrape on your body, there are a few things that happen in order to help you heal. The first step that happens after you cut yourself physically is that your body starts to go through hemostasis. This is the way that your body does what it can to stop the bleeding. At first, at this moment, your body is not concerned with healing. Your body is not going to immediately cover up that wound. All that matters are that the blood stops pouring out so that you don't have to lose any more of that.

This is incredibly powerful. This is what we do mentally. As soon as we experience something traumatic, our bodies will try to stop it. It doesn't try to heal. It doesn't try to make sense of what's going on, and it doesn't try to give us a deep explanation to help further establish what we have been through. The only thing that our body does at this moment is trying to make the trauma stop. It does whatever it can to make sure that we don't have to endure this pain anymore. Your body is incredibly powerful like this.

Understand what you might have gone through to make you try and stop the trauma. What experiences did you live through when your body did whatever it could to make this stop?

Did you try to self-sooth using outside sources? Maybe alcohol or drugs were able to stop the constant terror that ran through your mind.

Recognize this and remind yourself that whatever you have experienced is completely normal. This was your way your body tried to heal. We are past the stage now. Now it is time to move on.

After you get a cut and the bleeding has stopped, what occurs is inflammation. This inflammation is your body's way of fighting off any infection. It makes sure that the groundwork is in place for the actual restructuring of your skin to start.

Inflammation can be what occurs in us. This is when we are crying, when we are in pain, when we are screaming from anger, or when we are begging for things to stop. This is the stage that you might have gone through, but you are past this now. Your body was brave enough to pull you from this. You are so strong that you didn't have to deal with this anymore.

Your body did whatever it could to fight off this trauma and prevent it from happening again.

The point of this stage is to start a new growth process. You have moved past the initial fear and shock of what happened, and instead, you're looking for a way to heal. Unfortunately, not all of us understand the way that we are able to heal ourselves. This is when some things can get a little trickier. You are working through this now. You are fighting off this infection from ever coming back and taking over.

Proliferation. This is when the wound can start to close. Finally, it is not a sore spot anymore. This is the part that we need to focus on. You are focused on moving forward now. You understand that this wound is closing. It is finally healing. The skin is connected to itself once again to make sure that nothing can get in and nothing can get out.

Finally, in the stage of healing, your wound can form something new. This is when there might be a scar.

This is when you could be experiencing a reshaping of a physical part of your body. This is what happens to our soul. After we've experienced something traumatic, we never go back to the exact same way that things used to be. Instead, we only move forward and move on to something greater and better in the end.

Some people's wounds might heal incorrectly. They might let it become scar tissue on their soul, stopping another thing from functioning properly. You are not going to let this happen. You are healing now. You are feeling that wound finally close up. You don't have to let the feelings and emotions that you had at the time pour out anymore.

You're not closing things up so that you never deal with it again. You are simply closing it up because you are stronger and better now. You are moving past these challenging emotions. No longer do you have the challenging thoughts and feelings that used to pop up so frequently in the past.

The thing about scar tissue is that it will never be the same. Some scars will heal perfectly normally, and we don't even have to think about it. Then, there are plenty of other scars that can leave huge marks that can't be looked past. Eventually you'll get used to it. It is a part of you now, and this does not have to be so ugly. We don't have to consider scars as something scary or grotesque. They are simply another marking on our bodies. How many marks do you have simply from not even realizing that they are there?

Maybe there's a freckle on your cheek or a little cut on your arm from when you were a child and fell off your bike. Maybe you have some acne from when you were a teenager, struggling with the constant constellation of pimples across your face. Perhaps you can't grow hair on a certain patch on your body because of the scar. Maybe there's a big ugly lump on your leg that you hate to look at.

Whatever these are, we don't have to be afraid of them just like you don't have to fear the scar that is on your soul. You are moving on and past this now into a happier and healthier place. This scar is part of what makes you beautiful. Think of all the markings on a physical object that you see. Maybe you pull a little penny out of your change purse and notice all the small markings on this.

Chapter 3: Lose Weight Fast and Naturally

Numerous individuals are uncertain about how to lose weight securely and normally. It does not support that multiple sites and notices, especially those having a place with companies that sell diet drugs or other weight-loss products, promote misinformation about losing weight.

As indicated by 2014 research, a great many people who look for tips on the most proficient method to get thinner will go over false or deluding information on weight reduction.

"Fad" diets and exercise regimens can, at times, be hazardous as they can keep individuals from meeting their nourishing needs.

As indicated by the Centers for Disease Control and Prevention, the most secure measure of weight to lose every week is somewhere in the range of 1 and 2 pounds. The individuals who suffer substantially more every week or attempt craze diets or projects are significantly more prone to recover weight.

1. Keeping Refreshing Bites at Home and In the Workplace

Individuals frequently pick to eat nourishments that are helpful, so it is ideal to abstain from keeping prepackaged tidbits and confections close by.

One investigation found that individuals who kept unhealthful nourishment at home thought that it was increasingly hard to keep up or lose weight.

Keeping healthty snacks at home and work can enable an individual to meet their nourishing needs and maintain a strategic distance from an abundance of sugar and salt. Great snack choices include:

- Nuts with no added salt or sugar
- Natural products
- Prechopped vegetables
- Low-fat yoghurts
- Dried seaweed

2. Removing Processed Foods

Processed foods are high in sodium, fat, calories, and sugar. They frequently contain fewer supplements than entire nourishments.

As indicated by a primer research study, processed foods are substantially more likely than different food sources to prompt addictive eating practices, which will, in general outcome in individuals indulging.

3. Eating More Protein

An eating routine high in protein can enable an individual to lose weight. A diagram of existing examination on high protein eats fewer carbs inferred that they are an effective system for forestalling or treating obesity.

The information demonstrated that higher-protein diets of 25–30 grams of protein for each feast gave enhancements in hunger, bodyweight the board, cardiometabolic hazard components, or these wellbeing results.

- Fish
- Beans, peas, and lentils
- White poultry
- Low-fat cottage cheese
- Tofu

4. Stopping Included Sugar

Sugar is not in every case simple to maintain a strategic distance from; however, disposing of handled nourishments is a positive initial step to take.

As per the National Cancer Institute, men matured 19 years

and more established devour a normal of more than 19 teaspoons of included sugar a day. Ladies in a similar age bunch eat more than 14 teaspoons of added sugar a day.

A significant part of the sugar that individuals devour originates from fructose, which the liver separates and transforms into fat. After the liver converts the sugar into fat, it discharges these fat cells into the blood, which can prompt weight gain.

5. Drinking Black Coffee

Coffee may have some constructive wellbeing impacts if an individual forgoes, including sugar and fat. The writers of a survey article saw that coffee improved the body's processing of carbohydrates and fats.

A like look at featured a relationship between coffee utilization and a lower danger of diabetes and liver disease.

6. Remaining Hydrated

Water is the best liquid that an individual can drink for the day. It contains no calories and gives an abundance of health benefits.

At the point when an individual drinks water for the day, the water helps increment their digestion. Drinking water before a feast can likewise help decrease the sum that they eat.

At long last, if individuals supplant sweet refreshments with water, this will help decrease all outnumber of calories that they devour for the day.

7. Keeping Away from The Calories in Beverages

Soft drinks, natural product squeezes, and sports and caffeinated drinks regularly contain abundant sugar, which can prompt weight increase and make it progressively hard for an individual to get in shape.

Other high-calorie drinks incorporate liquor and strength espressos, like lattes, which contain milk and sugar.

Individuals can have a go at supplanting, at any rate, one of these drinks every day with water, shining water with lemon, or an herbal tea.

8. Avoiding Refined Carbohydrates

Proof in The American Journal of Clinical Nutrition recommends that refined sugars might be more harmful to the body's digestion than saturated fats.

Considering the convergence of sugar from refined starches, the liver will make and discharge fat into the circulatory system.

To diminish weight and keep it off, an individual can eat

entire grains.

Refined or simple carbohydrates incorporate the accompanying nourishments:

- White rice
- White bread
- White flour
- Candies
- Numerous sorts of cereal
- Included sugars
- Numerous sorts of pasta

Rice, bread, and pasta are, for the most part, accessible in entire grain varieties, which can help weight reduction and help shield the body from disease.

9. Fasting in Cycles

Fasting for short periods may enable an individual to get more fit. As per a recent report, irregular fasting or substitute day fasting can allow an individual to get in shape and keep up their weight reduction.

However, not every person should quick. Fasting can be dangerous for kids, creating adolescents, pregnant ladies, older individuals, and individuals with hidden wellbeing conditions.

10. Counting Calories and Keeping A Nourishment Diary

Counting calories can be a viable method to abstain from gorging. By tallying calories, an individual will know about precisely the amount they are devouring. This mindfulness can assist them with removing superfluous calories and settle on better dietary decisions.

A nourishment diary can enable an individual to consider what and the amount they are devouring each day. By doing this, they can likewise guarantee that they are getting enough of each stimulating nutrition type, for example, vegetables and proteins.

11. Brushing Teeth Between Dinners or Prior at Night

Notwithstanding improving dental cleanliness, brushing the teeth can help lessen the impulse to nibble between dinners.

If an individual who regularly snacks around evening time brushes their teeth prior at night, they may feel less enticed to eat extra snacks.

12. Eating More Fruits and Vegetables

An eating routine wealthy in products of the soil can enable an individual to get more fit and keep up their weight reduction.

The author of an orderly survey supports this case, expressing that advancing an expansion in products of the soil utilization is probably not going to cause any weight increase, even without instructing individuals to diminish their use regarding different nourishments.

13. Lessening Carbohydrate Consumption

Diets low in basic starches can enable an individual to reduce their weight by constraining the measure of added sugar that they eat.

Restorative low carbohydrate abstains from food center around expending entire sugars, high fats, fiber, and lean proteins. Rather than restricting all sugars for a brief period, this ought to be a reasonable, long haul dietary alteration.

14. Eating More Fiber

Fiber offers a few potential advantages to an individual hoping to get thinner. Research in Nutrition expresses that an expansion in fiber utilization can enable an individual to feel fuller more rapidly.

Furthermore, fiber helps weight reduction by advancing absorption and adjusting the microorganisms in the gut.

15. Expanding Traditional Cardiovascular and Resistance Training

Numerous individuals do not practice regularly and may likewise have inactive occupations. It is critical to incorporate both cardiovascular (cardio) work out, for example, running or strolling, and opposition preparing in a regular exercise program.

Cardio enables the body to consume calories rapidly while obstruction preparing manufactures fit bulk. Bulk can assist individuals with consuming more calories very still.

Furthermore, explore has discovered that individuals who take an interest in high-intensity interval training (HIIT) can lose more weight and see more prominent enhancements in their cardiovascular wellbeing than individuals who are utilizing other mainstream strategies for weight reduction.

16. Devouring Whey Protein

Individuals who use whey protein may expand their slender bulk while diminishing muscle versus fat, which can help with weight reduction.

Research from 2014 found that whey protein, in the mix with practice or a weight reduction diet, may help diminish body weight and muscle to fat ratio.

17. Eating Slowly

Eating slowly can enable an individual to decrease all outnumber of calories that they expend in one sitting. The purpose behind this is it can require some investment to understand that the stomach is full.

One examination showed that eating rapidly relates to corpulence. While the investigation couldn't prescribe mediations to enable an individual to eat all the more gradually, the outcomes do propose that eating nourishment at a slower pace can help decrease calorie consumption.

Biting nourishment completely and eating at a table with others may enable an individual to back off while eating.

18. Including Chili

Adding spice to nourishments may enable an individual to get more fit. Capsaicin is a compound that is normally present in flavors, for example, bean stew powder, and may have constructive outcomes.

For instance, inquire about demonstrates that capsaicin can assist ignite with fatting and increment digestion, yet at low rates.

19. Getting More Sleep

There is a link between corpulence and an absence of value

rest. The research proposes that getting adequate rest can add to weight loss. The researchers found that ladies who depicted their rest quality as poor or reasonable were more averse to effectively get in shape than the individuals who detailed their rest quality as being generally excellent.

20.   Utilizing a Smaller Plate

Utilizing smaller plates could have a positive mental impact. Individuals will, in general, fill their plate, so lessening the size of the plate may help decrease the measure of nourishment that an individual eats in one sitting. A 2015 systematic reassessment inferred that diminishing plate size could affect partition control and vitality utilization, yet it was hazy whether this was material over the full scope of bit sizes. Individuals hoping to get in shape securely and normally should concentrate on making a perpetual way of life changes instead of embracing brief measures.

Individuals must concentrate on making changes that they can keep up. Now and again, an individual may want to execute changes steadily or take a stab at presenting each in turn.

Chapter 4: Learning to Avoid Temptations and Triggers

While telling a person to adopt the traits of the mentally strong is a good way to develop mental toughness, it may not always be enough. In a way, it's a bit like telling a person that in order to be healthy you need to eat right, exercise, and get plenty of rest. Such advice is good and even correct, however, it lacks a certain specificity that can leave a person feeling unsure of exactly what to do. Fortunately, there are several practices that can create a clear plan of how to achieve mental toughness. These practices are like the actual recipes and exercises needed in order to eat right and get plenty of exercises. By adopting these practices into your daily routine, you will begin to develop mental toughness in everything you do and, in every environment, you find yourself in.

Keep Your Emotions in Check

The most important thing you can do in the quest for developing mental toughness is to keep your emotions in check. People who fail to take control of their emotions allow their emotions to control them. More often than not, this takes the form of people who are driven by rage, fear, or both. Whenever a person allows their emotions to control them, they allow their emotions to control their decisions, words, and actions. However, when you keep your emotions in check, you take control of your decisions, words, and actions, thereby taking control of your life overall.

In order to keep your emotions in check you have to learn to allow your emotions to subside before reacting to a situation. Therefore, instead of speaking when you are angry, or making a decision when you are frustrated, take a few minutes to allow your emotions to settle down. Take a moment to simply sit down, breathe deeply, and allow your energies to restore balance. Only when you feel calm and in control should you make your decision, speak your mind, or take any action.

Practice Detachment

Another critical element for mental toughness is what is known as detachment. This is when you remove yourself emotionally from the particular situation that is going on around you. Even if the situation affects you directly, remaining detached is a very positive thing. The biggest benefit of detachment is that it prevents an emotional response to the situation at hand. This is particularly helpful when things are not going according to plan.

Practicing detachment requires a great deal of effort at first. After all, most people are programmed to feel emotionally attached to the events going on around them at any given time. One of the best ways to practice detachment is to tell yourself that the situation isn't permanent. What causes a person to feel fear and frustration when faced with a negative situation is that they feel the situation is permanent. When you realize that even the worst events are temporary, you avoid the negative emotional response they can create.

Another way to become detached is to determine the reason you feel attached to the situation in the first place. In the case that someone is saying or doing something to hurt your feelings, understand that their words and actions are a reflection of them, not you. As long as you don't feed into their negativity you won't experience the pain they are trying to cause. This is true for anything you experience. By not feeding a negative situation or event with negative emotions, you prevent that situation from connecting to you. This allows you to exist within a negative event without being affected by it.

Accept What Is Beyond Your Control

Acceptance is one of the cornerstones of mental toughness. This can take the form of accepting yourself for who you are and accepting others for who they are, but it can also take the form of accepting what is beyond your control. When you learn to accept the things you can't change, you rewrite how your mind reacts to every situation you encounter. The fact of the matter is that the majority of stress and anxiety felt by the average person is the result of not being able to change certain things. Once you learn to accept those things you can't change, you eliminate all of that harmful stress and anxiety permanently.

While accepting what is beyond your control will take a little practice, it is actually quite easy in nature. The trick is to simply ask yourself if you can do anything at all to change the situation at hand. If the answer is 'no,' simply let it go. Rather than wasting time and energy fretting about what you can't control, adopt the mantra "It is what it is." This might seem careless at first, but after a while you will realize that it is a true sign of mental strength. By accepting what is beyond your control, you conserve your energy, thoughts, and time for those things you can affect, thereby making your efforts more effective and worthwhile.

Always Be Prepared

Another way to build mental toughness is to always be prepared. If you allow life to take you from one event to another, you will feel lost, uncertain, and unprepared for the experiences you encounter. However, when you take the time to prepare yourself for what lies ahead, you will develop a sense of being in control of your situation at all times. There are two ways to be prepared, and they are equally important for developing mental toughness.

The first way to be prepared is to prepare your mind at the beginning of each and every day. This takes the form of you taking time in the morning to focus your mind on who you are, what you are capable of, and your outlook on life in general. Whether you refer to this time as mediation, contemplation, or daily affirmations, the basic principle is the same. You simply focus your mind on what you believe and the qualities you aspire to. This will keep you grounded in your ideals throughout the day, helping you to make the right choices regardless of what life throws your way.

The second way to always be prepared is to take the time to prepare yourself for the situation at hand. If you have to give a presentation, make sure to give yourself plenty of time to prepare for it. Go over the information you want to present, choose the materials you want to use, and even take the time to make sure you have the exact clothes you want to wear. When you go into a situation fully prepared, you increase your self-confidence, giving you an added edge. Additionally, you will eliminate the stress and anxiety that results from feeling unprepared.

Take the Time to Embrace Success

One of the problems many negatively minded people experience is that they never take the time to appreciate success when it comes to their way. Sometimes they are too afraid of jinxing that success to actually recognize it. Most of the time, however, they are unable to embrace success because their mindset is simply too negative for such a positive action. Mentally strong people, by contrast, always take the time to embrace the successes that come their way. This serves to build their sense of confidence as well as their feeling of satisfaction with how things are going.

Following time, you experience a success of any kind, make sure you take a moment to recognize it. You can make an external statement, such as going out for drinks, treating yourself to a nice lunch, or some similar expression of gratitude. Alternatively, you can simply take a quiet moment to reflect on the success and all the effort that went into making it happen. There is no right or wrong way to embrace success, you just need to find a way that works for you. The trick to embracing success is in not letting it go to your head. Rather than praising your efforts or actions, appreciate the fact that things went well. Also, be sure to appreciate those whose help contributed to your success.

Be happy with what you have

Contentment is another element that is critical for mental toughness. In order to develop contentment, you have to learn how to be happy with what you have. This doesn't mean that you eliminate ambition or the desire to achieve greater success, rather it means that you show gratitude for the positives that currently exist. After all, the only way you will be able to truly appreciate the fulfillment of your dreams is if you can first appreciate your life the way it is.

One example of this is learning to appreciate your job. This is true whether you like your job or not. Even if you hate your job and desperately want to find another one, always take the time to appreciate the fact that you have a job in the first place. The fact is that you could be jobless, which would create all sorts of problems in your life. So, even if you hate your job, learn to appreciate it for what it is. This goes for everything in your life. No matter how good or bad a thing is, always appreciate having it before striving to make a change.

Be Happy with Who You Are

In addition to appreciating what you have, you should always be happy with who you are. Again, this doesn't mean that you should settle for who you are and not try to improve your life, rather it means that you should learn to appreciate who you are at every moment. There will always be issues that you want to fix in your life, and things you know you could do better. The problem is that if you focus on the things that are wrong, you will always see yourself in a negative light. However, when you learn to appreciate the good parts of your personality, you can pursue self-improvement with a sense of pride, hope, and optimism for who you will become as you begin to fulfill your true potential.

Chapter 5: Weight Loss Through Self Hypnosis

Hypnosis can stop those anomalous wants and noon sneaking into the kitchen. Overall, let us delve into the genuine meaning of hypnosis to build up realities in that impact. Hypnosis is a psychological state where you are in a stupor, where you are dependent upon recommendations, self-proposal, or autosuggestions. In hypnotherapy meetings, you are in hypnotic acceptance where you are increasingly responsive to new thoughts and orders since the mind is in an open state.

Is it extremely compelling? How can it work? Before whatever else, this is not enchantment. In contrast to the prevalent view, it cannot mysteriously reboot, reset, or reconstruct the human mind to accomplish results. It is a progression of outrageous fixation followed by unwinding and center that actuates the mind to redesign its eating propensities and hold them reliably. As per anderbilt edu, considers indicating weight loss because of hypnosis alone are very few and experience the ill effects of methodological issues. Some individuals suffered hypnosis for weight loss, and following 12 weeks, the damage a normal of 10.2lbs. The outcomes were promising and fascinating to the media, yet the benchmark group was little, and we cannot sum up the finding that it will be compelling to everybody.

The center of the hypnosis treatment for weight loss is to reinvent or change an individual's conduct towards nourishment, diet, and different variables that trigger weight loss. For instance, if one individual is inclined to binges on account of emotional eating, hypnosis can propose new responses. At the point when looked by a terrible day or nearly at the highest point of emotional eating, one can suggest that as opposed to venting out on dessert, one can go to the rec center and exercise.

Hypnosis results pass on that it is critical to realize that social change in relationship with weight the executives are unquestionably more essential and viable than hypnosis alone. You can ask your therapist or a hypnosis expert regarding this, yet before you submit on anything, talk with your doctor first. It is unequivocally recommended that you ensure the impacts of a changed eating example to your wellbeing. Here and there, eating designs are reactions to some hidden neurotic as well as dietary infirmities, for example, diabetes. For the individuals who have nourishment irregularity, be additional careful in putting your mind under hypnosis. Your wellbeing emphatically relies upon how and what you eat. Changing them implies putting your wellbeing needs undermined.

Traditionally, the main way individuals can accomplish weight loss is through sweating it off in the exercise center and essentially starving themselves in a diet that causes them to feel denied and testy. Today a lot of options and one of a kind strategy has been found to support dieters, and weight loss through hypnosis is one of these ways. Utilizing hypnosis to help accomplish weight loss works under the rule that weight loss starts with the mind. You can utilize your mind to control all that you do, and when allurements come to keep you off your track, your first and most grounded weapon to battle this enticement is your mind. Regardless of whether you inevitably win the weight loss fight through dieting and working out, having a prepared and taught mind could spell the distinction among progress and disappointment.

Weight loss through hypnosis considers the way that the mind is your most grounded weapon with regards to getting more fit, and this is the thing that it taps. Hypnosis is the point at which an individual is brought under a modified condition of cognizance, and it has been utilized for social examinations and purposes. A few people are recommending that a trance specialist can be tapped to spellbind the individual who is attempting to lose the weight and adjust key practices that will enable that individual to lose the weight. It is not necessarily the case that hypnosis will work essentially all alone. Despite what might be expected, weight loss through hypnosis is simply utilized as a device to make the ordinary techniques considerably progressively powerful.

Hypnosis along these lines is only a path for individuals to get an adjusted mental cognizance concerning how they see their excursion. This is just powerful whenever taken together with a compelling project. By the day's end, shedding pounds is tied in with practicing normally and satisfactorily, just as controlling the sort and the measure of nourishment that you eat. These dietary limitations and exercise necessities need a ton of control and resolution, and this is the place hypnosis comes in. You cannot win your fight with overabundance weight without enough resolution, because the fight starts with the mind. Self-discipline influences how solid you are in observing your weight loss program through to the end.

What Does Weight Loss Through Hypnosis Take?

Getting More Fit Is an Included Procedure

A lot should be tended to and changed to get more fit. No incredible new data for you there. In any case, did you realize that by utilizing weight loss through hypnosis, you could make that procedure simpler and increasingly pleasurable? You can make it a programmed foolish procedure that, when you remain with it, will bring you down to a significantly more alluring and attractive weight. In the following couple of seconds, I will give you one of the manners in which you can do this.

You have presumably been on diets previously and battled to keep up a prohibitive diet. Furthermore, what occurs? At the point when somebody, even you, reveals to you that you cannot eat a specific nourishment, that nourishment turns out to be much progressively attractive. You begin to want that specific nourishment, not because you need it, but since you cannot have it. These prohibitive projects additionally have another drawback. When you confine your nourishment admission to too scarcely any calories, your body, through an endurance instrument, thinks there is starvation and begins to hinder your digestion from moderating your vitality stores—the exact inverse of what you need to occur if you are attempting to get in shape. So prohibitive diets do not work. It is simply that basic.

Furthermore, if you've at any point been on a tight eating routine, you most likely saw this as obvious. You restored all the weight when you quit eating in that prohibitive way. Things can be distinctive when you use weight loss through hypnosis.

Things being what they are, by what method can weight loss through hypnosis improve this procedure?

At the point when you are entranced, something that an accomplished and very much prepared subliminal specialist will have the option to do is to change your reaction to nourishment and eating. We are brought into the world with the best possible conduct toward nourishment that we need to have. That conduct is to eat when hungry and stop when full. Have you, at any point, see how a newborn child eats? A baby eats until it is full and afterward stops. It lets out the areola and will eat because it need not bother with the nourishment any longer. It has provided itself with the fundamental supplements it requires to deal with its requirements for the following couple of hours.

Recapturing the Apparatuses Given You During Childbirth

You were brought into the world with that equivalent capacity. A very much prepared trance inducer can make the states that are essential for you to make changes in your reactions and responses to foods... even the contemplations of nourishment. Furthermore, by doing only this straightforward procedure, you begin to see nourishment and eating unexpectedly. You are never again constrained by nourishment. You are happy with a limited quantity of nourishment. You recover power over the straightforward undertaking of providing supplements to your body, and that feels better.

This is only one of the techniques that are utilized in helping you recapture command over nourishment and shed pounds utilizing hypnosis for weight loss.

So, if you need to encounter weight loss through hypnosis to assist you with losing weight, something you need is to make the state where nourishment is simply one more item that we use to supply life, such as breathing and drinking water. You can move nourishment out of your awareness with the goal that it is the thing that it was proposed to be, a characteristic component like air, utilized for supporting life.

Weight Loss through Hypnosis - Hype or Not

Consistently, you are shelled with new items out in the market, guaranteeing that such and such an item can assist you with shedding 10 pounds in about fourteen days or assist you with being a skinnier individual in only one month. Have you ever caught wind of weight loss through hypnosis? There are a lot of surveys been done about this procedure. Some surveys offered go-ahead for hypnosis, and there are some who scrutinized its validity and the fundamental motivation behind why an individual can shed pounds through it.

Is it enchantment, or is it a logical truth? Weight loss through hypnosis may sound persuading; however, accomplishes it truly work? Like some other weight loss program or item, everything relies upon the distinct individual. One may work for you and not for your companion. This new thought of hypnosis comparable to weight loss has been given accentuation while contemplates have uncovered that the individuals who have experienced the procedure without a doubt lose the weight and even kept it up after some time.

The mystery? Your mind. The mind is ground-breaking to such an extent that it very well may be the way to helping you lose those pounds you constantly needed to lose. You can discover CDs that contain a few projects that can help you in molding your brain and oversee your life.

You can get data on the how-to and the things expected to make weight loss through hypnosis like how to supplant undesirable propensities with sound ones, how to check your longings and be in charge rather than your weight controlling your life. These CDs contain portrayal and guidelines. It resembles somebody is conversing with you, in a quieting voice while inspiring you to carry on with a solid way of life while getting in shape. It resembles having a companion who can help you when you are at an intersection in your life.

The mind can do it can wreck or improve your life. Everything happens directly inside your mind. At the point when you know how to control your desires, inspire yourself, or be taught in arriving at your objective, then certainly you will have the body you constantly needed for the long haul.

Chapter 6: Daily Guided Meditation Techniques

3 Minutes Guided Meditation

Sit comfortably in a cross-legged posture

If you are not comfortable sitting in a cross-legged posture, position yourself on a chair

Keep your back straight

You can use a backrest but not a headrest

Close your eyes comfortably

Start breathing normally

Breathe in slowly

Let the air enter through your nostrils

Feel the warmth of the air as it enters

Fill your lungs with the air

Feel it entering your abdomen

Hold your breath for a few moments

Now, release the breath slowly through your mouth

Breathe in slowly

Hold your breath

Breathe out

Thoughts may start entering your mind

Pay no attention to them

If your attention is getting diverted

Simply observe the thoughts but don't get involved

Focus on your breathing

Breathe in

Breathe out

If you are getting distracted

Breathe in and count backward from 4

4...3...2...1

Hold your breath to the count backward from 4

4...3...2...1

Release your breath slowly backward to the count of 7

7...6...5...4...3...2...1

Repeat this process 3 times

Breathe in and count backward from 4

4...3...2...1

Hold your breath to the count backward from 4

4...3...2...1

Release your breath slowly backward to the count of 7

7...6...5...4...3...2...1

Every exhalation takes away stress and negativity

Breathe in and count backward from 4

4...3...2...1

Hold your breath to the count backward from 4

4...3...2...1

Release your breath slowly backward to the count of 7

7...6...5...4...3...2...1

You are feeling good, there is nothing disturbing you

Breathe in and count backward from 4

4...3...2...1

Hold your breath to the count backward from 4

4...3...2...1

Release your breath slowly backward to the count of 7

7...6...5...4...3...2...1

You are calm and relaxed now

Your mind would get settled and the thoughts wouldn't disturb you

Now start breathing normally and become aware of your surroundings

Open your eyes gently

5 Minutes Guided Meditation

Sit comfortably in a cross-legged posture

If you are not comfortable sitting in a cross-legged posture, position yourself on a chair

Keep your back straight

You can use a backrest but not a headrest

Close your eyes comfortably

Start breathing normally

Breathe in slowly

Let the air enter through your nostrils

Feel the warmth of the air as it enters

Fill your lungs with the air

Feel it entering your abdomen

Hold your breath for a few moments

Now, release the breath slowly through your mouth

Breathe in slowly

Hold your breath

Breathe out

Thoughts may start entering your mind

Pay no attention to them

If your attention is getting diverted

Simply observe the thoughts but do not get involved

Focus on your breathing

Breathe in

Breathe out

If you are getting distracted

Breathe in and count backward from 4

4...3...2...1

Hold your breath to the count backward from 4

4...3...2...1

Release your breath slowly backward to the count of 7

7...6...5...4...3...2...1

Your mind became calm

Your body release any tension

Repeat this process 3 times

Breathe in and count backward from 4

4...3...2...1

Hold your breath to the count backward from 4

4...3...2...1

Release your breath slowly backward to the count of 7

7...6...5...4...3...2...1

Breathe in and count backward from 4

4...3...2...1

Hold your breath to the count backward from 4

4...3...2...1

Release your breath slowly backward to the count of 7

7...6...5...4...3...2...1

Breathe in and count backward from 4

4...3...2...1

Hold your breath to the count backward from 4

4...3...2...1

Release your breath slowly backward to the count of 7

7...6...5...4...3...2...1

Now, look at the thoughts in your mind

Become aware of those thoughts

Simply observe them from a distance

Do not take part in them

Do not judge these thoughts

Simply observe the kind of thoughts originating in your mind

They do not concern you now

You do not need to react to these thoughts

Simply become aware of them

Once you become fully aware of these thoughts, they will stop affecting you

Do not run from these thoughts

Accept and embrace them

Bring your attention to your bringing

It is the most important thing now

Breathe in

Hold your breath

Breathe out

Breathe in

Hold your breath

Breathe out

You are very calm and aware

Breathe in

Hold your breath

Breathe out

You are feeling calm and relaxed now

There is no rush

No anxiety

No stress

No anger

No judgment

There is complete calm

Now start breathing normally and become aware of your surroundings

Open your eyes gently

7 Minute Guided Meditation

Take your position at the place of your meditation

Be seated

Sit in a completely relaxed manner

Do not do anything immediately

Ground yourself first

Just sit completely relaxed for a few minutes

Get into a comfortable position

Keep your back straight

Ensure that your shoulders are also straight

Your back and neck should be in a straight line

Now, close your eyes

Lean slightly forward and then backward

Lean-to your left side and then to your right

Now, bring yourself to the center and find the best and most comfortable position

Feel your head positioned on your neck

Raise your chin slightly upwards

This will help you in placing your focus between your eyebrows

Try to feel your whole body

Notice if there is tension anywhere

If you feel any part tense, release the tension

Adjust your body to release the pressure

Now start breathing normally

Inhale through your nose

Exhale through your mouth

Take short inhalations

Hold your breath for a few seconds

Exhale through your mouth longer

Breathe in

Breathe out

Breathe in

Breathe out

Breathe in

Breathe out

Now, focus on the air you are breathing

Feel the warmth of this air

Trace the path taken by the air in your body

Watch it entering your lungs

Feel the expansion of your chest

Feel your stomach getting inflated

Hold your breath for a few seconds now

Count till 4

1....2....3....4

Now, exhale slowly through your mouth

Exhale for the count of 7

1....2....3....4......5....6....7

Again, repeat the process

Inhale to the count of 4

1....2....3....4

Feel it entering your body

Hold your breath for a few seconds now

Count till 4

1....2....3....4

Now, exhale slowly through your mouth

Exhale for the count of 7

1....2....3....4......5....6....7

You are feeling relaxed now

As you exhale you drive away from the negative thoughts and emotions

You are breathing in positivity

Smile as you breathe every time

Feel relaxed as you exhale

This relaxation is natural

It is the natural state of your body

Your body is designed to remain in a relaxed state

You are working to bring it into its natural state

Do not be bothered by your thoughts and emotions

Thoughts will come into your mind

There is no need to worry about them

The harder you will try to push them

The more aggressive they will get

You must embrace and accept them

You should not get affected by them

You should not judge them

Simply observe them from a distance

Like someone observes the traffic on the road standing in the balcony

The traffic is not a problem for that person

It is still there

But that person is not stuck in it

For his, those are some cars standing behind each other

There is no inconvenience

In the same way, these thoughts should also not be a problem for you

They should invoke no reaction

You are not involved in them actively

You are simply observing their creation and futility

You are not interested in them

They cannot affect you

You are getting bored with them

Bring back your focus to your breathing

Inhale slowly

Watch your chest rise as the air fills your lungs

Watch your stomach inflate as air enters it

Hold your breath for a few seconds

Pressure is building

Now slowly exhale

All the pressure inside you will go away with the breath

You are feeling light with every exhale

You are feeling great

This is an amazingly liberating feeling

Repeat the process again

Breathe in

Hold the breath

Exhale slowly

Now your mind is getting clear

You are feeling relaxed

There are no worries

There is no stress

You are feeling light

Focus once again on your breath

Inhale deeply

Let the air enter your body freely

Let it take its own course

Simply follow the path the air takes

Hold it for a few seconds

Now observe the remaining stress going out with the breath

Now start breathing normally

Stabilize your breathing

Let it return to its normal rate

Remain seated with your eyes closed

Try to feel your surrounding

You are feeling very relaxed now

You can open your eyes.

Chapter 7: Background Information for Weight Loss

Understand Your Habits

You may find yourself developing some habits without knowing. The same applies to create excellent health practice. Your daily practices and choices explain your current conditions. Stop complaining; do focus on your habits, remember your preferences will define who you will be. Albert Einstein goes on to say, "we cannot solve our problems with the same thinking we used when we created them." Step out of your bubble a given structure for the desired outcome. Really the hardest part is starting, and you've already done that, and it will only get more accessible and more natural the more you participate and the more you take an active role in this journey.

Consider habits development as elaborated in the story of a Miller and a camel on a winter day. It was freezing outside, and while the miller was asleep, he was awakened by some noise on the door. Upon opening his eyes, he heard the voice of a camel complaining that it was cold outside and was requesting to warm his nose inside. Miller agreed that he was only to insert the nozzle. A little later, the camel put his forehead then the neck, then other parts of the body than the whole-body bit by bit until he started destroying things inside. He started walking in the house, stumbling on anything on its way. When the miller ordered the camel to move out, the came boasted that he was comfortable inside and would not leave. The camel went further to tell the miller that he could leave at his pleasure. The same goes for a habit that comes knocking about and taking over.

Maybe you started out smoking your first cigarette, thinking it was disgusting, and then years go by, and you have a nasty habit. Well, bad habits can sneak in, but the same philosophy can apply to ethical practices. Just take it bit by bit and step by step, and before you know it, you have healthy habits in your life. There are so many challenges to healthy eating. You have to be willing to have an open mind and reset your thinking on food.

It is cheaper to develop new habits; effort is the primary requirement, but not that much. When you have trained yourself new patterns, train on it every day for some time, after which it will be automatic.

We can relate that situation to a football club Coash who engages in various rigorous training with his players while awaiting the actual match. They practice new skills and moves. When match day arrives, the coach sits with the substitutes while watching the players playing from the line. Players play as per the learned skills and moves. Apply the required effort to actualize your goal.

While storying with your workmates, tell them how you drink 3 to for four glasses of water every day, the same as tea. That looks strict. In heart, you know how your consumption of water and team is reduced while at home. This is self-discipline. Self-discipline calls for the establishment of strong foundations. Efforts adopted is less.

Apply Core solutions

Recognize and face the challenges of healthy eating and develop new habits. Like a logger trying to clear a log, identify the critical side of each situation. The well-experienced logger will try to identify essential joints by climbing up then do the clearing. A less experienced logger would start by the edge. Both methods produce expected results, but one way saves more time and uses less energy than the other. All our problems have strategic points. How about when we identify critical logs to healthy eating and offer some solutions. First, log jam. How you were brought up. You may have been forced as a child to eat vegetables and see it as something undesirable, and you built a perception that plants don't taste good. Another log jam is stress. So much pressure.

We live in a world full of pressure where time matters in all our undertakings, troubled life, and our body pay most of the price. You have many choices to pick from. If you are a lover of fast food, you need to stop. Fast foods are addictive, and we highly depend on them due to the positive attitude we have towards them. We are obsessed with them such that we cannot live a day without consuming them. When you eat something wrong for you and you say, you don't care. Your thoughts and focus are totally on how delicious and enjoyable it is to be eating the food that you're eating, regardless of how unhealthy it is, and then you have guilt about how those pounds are going on rather than coming off.

Such thoughts occur even when taking tasty food. We may find ourselves eating some food which in reality we know are very dangerous to our health. Chip is a prime example. An individual from a diet class may feel hungry on her way back home and decide to a branch by a fast food joint for some plates of chips. Despite several cautions on the dangers of chips from class lessons, she chooses to eat chips—what a radical idea. Most people have mental disorders making it difficult to stop taking some food even though we understand their repercussions on our bodies. i.e., eating chips. An article on this topic claims that most food companies are working hard at night to make fast food more addictive. According to Howard Moskovitz, a consultant in the junk food industry, they put more flavor on junk food to make you come back for more. If the food tastes too good, then we'd have what's called a sensory-specific Satia T then we wouldn't want anymore. So, companies have to find just the right balance of flavors. So, there's not too much or too little. All they do is to balance the flavors. That balance is called Bliss point.

According to Steven Weatherly, an expert in junk food, Cheetos are the core source of pleasure. They are the specific type of food manufactured by big companies to solely satisfy you and not to add any health benefit to your body. They are designed in such a manner that when you start eating them, it melts on your mouth, making it feels tasty and impressive. They are made to make you go for more. A friend was once a diet, and her boyfriend brought home Cheetos. Yes, she said no. She ended up just having one, and before she knew it, she knew almost the whole thing. Now we understand why the next log in our way we maybe think we don't like healthy food. Perhaps you don't like healthy food. You want foods that excite your palate to feel alive, be closer to something exciting, but you will not be satisfied.

You'll not reach the maximum point, and perhaps you will not know what to do. Normalizing bad habits make us feel comfortable in our negative thoughts. When you do one negative thing, the effects widely spread. Self-indulgence keeps us wrapped up in this safe place and keeps us inside of ourselves and absorbed by negative thoughts. You know, you do one thing poorly or negatively, it trickles into other areas. It leaves you feeling bad, and you do short to feel better just for the short term, such as impossible diets that you can't keep up with, and then you, you feel worse and worse about yourself and you, you go overboard when you can't keep up. It's a vicious cycle. The primary method of overcoming these key log is to fist, hit the reset button. It might not be easy, strive as much as you can by having an open mind and a positive attitude going forward.

Explore various flavors even if you don't like them. Michael's sister has a negative attitude towards blueberries. She had not consumed any since her childhood and kept telling stories that had no connection to the blueberries' taste. One day Michael made her taste the blueberry, and she loved it. Test your assumptions, test your opinions because you don't know where they came from; such an assumption may be baseless. Despite her premise on blueberries being messy, and she made a try, and she ended up loving it. Open your mind for new ideas. Remember the story of the coy and to keep figuratively throwing yourself in more significant environments, you will stretch out and grow in size. Adopt an attitude of success and stop to fetus thinking and know that your thoughts, perceptions, and behaviors can change. Why not start to look forward to fruiting and vegetables, however crazy they sound? You were not born with thoughts you possess today; they are a construct of your mind. They can be challenged.

The next solution calls for changing one's health. Saying a big NO and breaking a cycle is all you need—cutting out indulgence.

Commit yourself daily, and you'll find it easier to overcome the notion of food industries that want you to be addicted to their food. The third is growth towards what you want and the freedom you desire. This step calls for exceptional consistency. Make your bold step a pattern. This pattern will develop into the desired habit. Unpack your true self through spiritual faith and meditative silence. Strive to become better. Look inside, stop looking for solutions on the outside. Make additional efforts like being more helpful to those that are happy and caring for those that are needy, consistently reach for truth, grace, and peace in your day. Take caution on being a man of the people, and you may be living a fishy life. Finally, systems generate autonomy. We are going to be creating a system together by planning, keeping it simple, embracing balance in your life, and accomplishing these solutions and your goals by following the system to help you prioritize and reinforce consistency in your life.

The best solution to weight loss is a healthy diet and an active body. There could be a reason why doing these two is a problem from your side. The pathway will make the process more holistic and more fun. All may not be your answer, but you must get something from it.

Chapter 8: Your PossibleWeight Loss Block

What beliefs are holding onto your weight?

I am inferior

I am lacking

I am inconsequential, so I have to make myself big to be seen

Losing weight is too difficult

I will fail and put the weight all back on again

I must be so awful and bad not to be able to control my eating

I want to punish myself

It is too hard to start dieting

My weight is ancestral, and I can't change that

My weight is genetic, and I can't change that

I am not good enough/I am not enough

I self-sabotage myself

I am worthless

I loathe myself

Healing negative beliefs

The best ways to heal negative beliefs and build confidence are: Emotional Freedom Technique (EFTTM)–Bach Flower Remedies Affirmations

Ask your guides and angels to help heal you. A pattern is a program that you have, which is part of your personality. For example, in your personality could be the thoughts:

I am not good enough

I am useless

I can't lose weight

I am not as good as other people

I am stupid

I am ugly

I am fat (remember if you tell yourself you are fat, you will be!)

I am to blame

It is my fault

I can't do anything right

I am a failure

This means that you block your weight loss as you feel that the task is too daunting, and you will fail. New patterns can be easily installed using EFTTM.

A block is something that stops you moving forward and the biggest one of these is FEAR. The other one is being safe. If your subconscious feels that it is not safe it WILL NOT LET YOU DO IT. So, if your subconscious feels that losing weight is not safe, you WILL NOT LOSE WEIGHT!

Also, if you think you are worthless or you feel you do not deserve, this will cause you to self-sabotage.

Healing negative patterns and blocks

The best ways to heal negative patterns and blocks are:

Emotional Freedom Technique

Bach Flower Remedies

Affirmations

Meditation

Ask your guides and angels to help heal you

What is self-sabotage?

The term, self-sabotage, describes our often-unconscious ability to stop ourselves being, doing or having; being the person we want to be, doing what we want to experience or achieve or having our goals and desires become a reality. Most of the time, we are totally unaware that we are self-sabotaging as it happens on a subconscious level. However, sometimes we are aware of that little voice in the back of our head that says, "you can't learn a language" or "don't be ridiculous, you can't lose weight."

Our subconscious mind is a powerful tool and always thinks that it is acting in our best interest. Stopping us stepping into new territory, discouraging us from taking risks ensures that we don't get hurt, we are not humiliated, and we don't fail, that is why so many projects never get off the ground. Rather than playing to win, self-sabotage plays to avoid defeat.

The purpose of this aspect of the subconscious is self-protection and survival. It can even negatively affect your health if it thinks that this will protect you from greater risk. Layers of excess weight have long been recognized as protection and very often the subconscious will use weight gain to protect you from perceived dangers you might be exposed to as a slimmer person.

For example, where someone has been abused as a child, the subconscious may add weight to make them unattractive (it thinks) so that the abuse is never repeated.

So, people may talk about self-sabotage in regard to their weight because they eat emotionally and put on weight. However, sometimes self-sabotage will affect your hormones and/or organs, causing weight gain in people who eat only a modest amount. Sometimes people can lose weight but always put it back on just another method of self-sabotage. Once the perceived need to protect through self-sabotage has been healed and released, our illnesses and weight may disappear.

My experience of self-sabotage

In my personal quest to lose the weight and water I had accumulated, I consulted a lady who specialized in 'muscle testing.' When we asked the question "Do I want to be slim," the clear reply was "no!" which took me totally by surprise. So then started the journey of discovery as to why my subconscious didn't want me to be slim.

Why was I self-sabotaging?

During the long seventeen years in which I slowly cleared and healed the reasons for my self- sabotage:

I had set up a self-punishment/self-destruct program because of what I had done in past lives

I had set up a protection around me (weight and water) because of the sexual abuse, date rape and male attention I had. I didn't feel it was safe to be a woman

I had several past life issues with starving to death and didn't want to starve in this lifetime

I had several past life issues with dying of thirst, hence the excess water in this lifetime to ensure that it didn't happen again

I had a tremendous amount of other karma

I thought that if I became a therapist I could not trust myself not to hurt, or experiment on patients, as I had hurt them before in past lives and so I was only going to be a therapist when I was 'slim'

I was frightened to take herbs as I had seen so many people die from them in past lives

Because I had been persecuted in past lives for healing people, I thought I would be persecuted in this life as well

I was frightened of being powerful

I was frightened to do the work I was supposed to do

I was frightened that the book would fail

Although I relate to my self-sabotage with weight and health there were many other areas of my life that affected.

I was always in debt and could never pay off my credit cards

I never got the job I deserved and was very often out of work

If I got a job, there would always be someone giving me a tough time (karmic payback!)

When I had any treatments, such as red vein treatment or plastic surgery, it would always go wrong

Believe it or not, my subconscious was creating a reality where all of the above occurred, the subconscious is that strong, believe me. Even when I had released the attachments, and got rid of the influence of my mother, my subconscious was still following their examples and as I strived to get better, my subconscious really kicked in and made it worse.

So, my subconscious was actually affecting all my organs and making them work inefficiently so that I put on six stone and swelled up with water. This was because my subconscious knew I could lose weight and it decided this was the best plan of attack.

That's why some people lose weight and then put it back on. The subconscious doesn't always realize what is happening to begin with, hence the weight loss. It then kicks in big time in survival mode and the weight goes back on. You would not lose six stone and then put it back on again, you might put back a stone and then get it off. People blame diets or losing it too quickly but, in fact, it is simply your subconscious sabotaging you.

Emotional and comfort eating

When you read magazine articles they always talk about emotional eating and weight gain. Some people do eat for emotional reasons and boredom. Some people do overeat and there are explanations for this. You need to identify your emotional eating triggers and use a technique such as EFTtm to eliminate them. However, if you want to eat, try to wait for a 10-minute period breathing deeply and you should find that after that, the need to eat has gone.

However, I know a lot of slim people who overeat and drink too much. They overeat for emotional reasons as well, slim people aren't perfect or without their own problems.

Overweight people do not eat emotionally any more than slim/normal people. How often are you on holiday and you watch people eat an enormous breakfast, followed by an enormous lunch and then three courses for dinner, plus booze, every day for two weeks? How often do you see a slim person eat a packet of biscuits or a bar of chocolate? ALL THE TIME!

You have to find the reasons why your subconscious doesn't want to lose weight and either release the reasons if these are past lives based or change your subconscious 'belief system' if they are more personality traits.

Removing the self-sabotage

When I was spending a huge amount of money with therapists and nothing worked, I did mention that I might be self-sabotaging myself. Most of them threw their hands up in horror and told me it was just an excuse to overeat (here we go again, I thought).

I read a lot about Emotional Freedom Technique (EFTTM) and in the very first paragraph, I read it mentioned self-sabotage. This was quite amazing. However, my self-sabotage was so deeply ingrained that for a long time, EFTTM just made everything worse, as my subconscious tried to hold onto its control of me.

I, therefore, had to dig much deeper by clearing the attachments, past lives, and karma and then I could use EFTTM and my other techniques to change my subconscious perception and its belief system that "I did not deserve."

Psychological reversal

I thought I wanted to lose weight, but I actually didn't and my subconscious was stopping me. You need to find out all the reasons why and release and heal them one by one. For this, you use the EFTTM psychological reversal techniques.

How are you self-sabotaging because my experience would lead me to believe that you are?

Habit of self-sabotage

I had a spiritual reading session and was told that the self-punishment had been healed but that I still had the 'habit' and that needed to be healed and not recreated. Our body and subconscious sabotage us so much that it becomes automatic and then a habit. So even when the original stimuli are healed, the habit remains. So, remember to test to see whether there is a habit and then heal accordingly (normally the same way you healed the original pattern).

Make sure you don't recreate the habit by repeating affirmations and if you feel yourself slipping back into 'deserving the pattern' immediately cancel this feeling and ensure that you keep healing it.

Chapter 9: The Importance of Genetics

How You Were Raised, Counts

Those who have been overweight all their lives go through certain cycles. There is a period of unhealthy habits, the recognition that there needs to be a change, an attempt at reform, the failure to follow through, and then back to a period of unhealthy habits. This cycle is present in many people that are overweight, but for those that were overweight kids and teens, it might be better understood. We might have also adopted this unhealthy cycle from our parents. Once we've found ourselves in this dangerous position, it can feel like clawing our way out when we decide we want to lose weight. If the pattern of behavior is not at first recognized, then we won't be able to determine the best method of breaking this unhealthy habit.

Studies have proven that kids who were weight-shamed go through cycles of binge eating and meal skipping that leads to self-loathing. A child that experiences criticism from their parents will start learning unhealthy methods of coping with weight and dieting. Eating is something that we've been doing all our lives, so the way that we eat now is undoubtedly related to the way that we used to be taught to eat. Parents that might have body-shamed their kids by telling them they needed to lose weight or stop eating so much are responsible for causing self-loathing later in life.

Weight-shaming is not just blatantly telling someone that they are fat. It might also cloud diet encouragement. If your mom or dad always told you to try out a diet or suggested that you shouldn't eat a particular food, which was probably enough for you to feel a certain amount of shame about your weight. Even having a parent that continually talks about dieting is likely to make a child feel as though they should diet, too.

Many kids might grow up with moms who are always trying out new diets and fads. By seeing this is a kid, we end up going through the same phases. Maybe a parent was always saying things like, "I need to start my diet on Monday." This idea gets it in the kid's head that diets are something they should aim for, but only at a moment of convenience. The way a parent or even older sibling always talked about their body will play into how you might see your own body now. Perhaps your mom was still saying things like, "I hate my thighs; they are so big!" If a girl looks in the mirror and sees she has the same shaped thighs as her mother, she'll end up thinking about how both she and her mother see those thighs as significant, even though the mother never said anything directly to the girl about her body.

It is challenging because most parents think they are helping. Parents that stock the fridge with Diet Coke instead of regular might think they are doing everyone a favor when really, they are still supplying a form of addiction. Those that make sure to weigh their kids or track their workout routines could be doing so just because they want to make sure their kid is healthy. Still, they might not realize they are setting them up in a fearful manner in which dieting and exercising are an authoritative issue. Parents who are strict with routines might raise kids that don't have any method at all as an act of rebellion.

How our parents' diet, exercise, and talk about health, in general, will also form our body perceptions. A daughter of a mother who consistently crashes diets and works out too hard will likely produce a daughter that does the same. A father that only eats microwave meals or fast food is setting his kids up for doing the same when they become adults. When this happens, it is an insidious issue that we might not even recognize. The things our parents do can seem normal to us, as it is behavior that we learn is standard.

Be mindful of how you talk about exercise around children. Whether they are your kids or someone else's, never talk about body issues around kids. If you walk around talking about how much you hate your belly flab, you are teaching the kids around you to evaluate their stomachs, wondering if they, too, have too much belly flab. Kids will be confronted with these body issues in other ways, as it is inevitable. As parents, caretakers, or any role models, we should be teaching our kids how to love their bodies and adequately take care of them because they deserve to be healthy, not because they should be skinnier or prettier.

Pregnant Moms Who Exercise Will Likely Give Birth to Healthy Kids

A study was conducted in which one group of pregnant rats were given exercise wheels, while another group of pregnant rats wasn't assigned anything. Those who used the exercise wheels ended up giving birth to more active babies. The babies of the moms that didn't work out would sit around and not do anything, as opposed to the babies of the moms that were always using an exercise wheel, who would use the wheel themselves. This was true for at least half of the rats born from active mothers. They weren't given anything else, so there weren't any factors to determine the difference in the level of activity other than the environment in which they were raised in the womb.

This exercise was inspired by similar research done on humans, though many scientists wonder if the effects were just because of a mother's influence after birth. Instead of assuming that it was from active pregnancy, many scientists speculate that the difference in the amount of desire for physical activity is because mothers with active pregnancies are also mothers with busy lives. Their lifestyle and habits can affect children, but the study with the rats proves that it might be on a level different than just the learned behavior.

Even in the womb, our mothers are teaching us how to exercise. We learn before we're also walking how vital exercise is in maintaining a high level of physical activity. If a mother is more active while she's pregnant, she's setting her unborn baby up for a future in which it is just generally more productive. This means that not only are we affected by the learned habits of our parents, but how we are actually created and grown also determines how much physical activity we let into our life.

Look back on your mother, father, or any other person that helped raise you, biologically or not. Were they active? Did they let that level of activity negatively affect your life? Did they reject exercise and healthy eating at all costs? Did you learn your unhealthy eating habits, or are they just a product of not being taught anything at all? We are taught how to eat and exercise, which means we are also taught how not to eat healthily or use. We can't entirely blame our parents for the way we live now, but it is still essential to recognize as it'll help bring us closer to closure with the unhealthy person in our head.

This is the right motivation for any woman hoping to get pregnant in the future. Starting a family is a goal for many different people. An essential aspect of starting that family is making sure to have a high level of physical activity. Kids require a lot of chasing and lifting. It is much harder for those that are not in shape to look after and give proper attention to active kids. It is also essential to be healthy when pregnant with them to get them started right away with a healthy lifestyle. After kids are born, parents are also responsible for making sure their kids understand how to live a healthy lifestyle that does not include any bad habits.

Chapter 10: How to Eat Right with The Help of Meditation

Eat fruits

When was the last time you went to the market with the intention of specifically buying fruits? You find that we purchase all other types of food, but we barely think of buying fruits. The good thing about fruits is that they are healthy, and they have plenty of nutritious benefits. If you are the type of person that loves sweet things, fruits can act as a good replacement. When consumed, they add value to your body and can prevent you from acquiring some diseases. Fruits also contain some minerals that are essential to your body. Now the question we have at the moment is how mediation will help you in taking the fruits. One of the benefits of meditating is that it allows you to differentiate between right and wrong. Eating fruits is beneficial to your body, and hence it is a good move to take.

Avoid processed foods

Currently, we are having a lot of processed foods. The food industry has been one of the fastest-growing industries. As the industry expands, the market becomes competitive, and more people join the industry. We are having new foods being introduced to the market as companies look forward to growing and gaining recognition. One of the common factors among all the companies is that they aim at pleasing the consumers. After carefully studying the target market, they know what each individual requires, which helps them in the production of their various items. If they are targeting a market with low purchasing power, they make products that are cheap and enticing. Some of the processed foods made by such companies contain a lot of chemicals and have harmful effects on the individual. You find that such foods are not helpful and only result in harm. These are the types of foods that we need to avoid if we wish to have good health. One of the things that you require for you to avoid such foods is discipline. It allows you to make the right decisions regarding what you consume, and you only take in what is helpful.

Avoid carbohydrates

In every meal that you take, you only require a small portion of carbohydrates. In most cases, we do the contrary and have the biggest percentage of our meal as a carbohydrate. When we go to this, our body receives more that it can utilize. One of the main purposes of consuming carbohydrates is that they provide us with energy. When they are consumed in excess, not all can be used to provide energy. The excess can be turned into fatty tissues, and one ends up adding some weight. In some cases, the carbohydrates can result in some diseases like cardiovascular diseases. To avoid weight gain and such diseases, it is better if one avoids taking large amounts of carbohydrates. Ensure that you only take the recommended portions. You also find that some of these foods, like bread, contain certain addictive substances. In the process, all you want to do is keep wanting to take more. As a result, you take up more than your body needs, and the excess does not benefit it in any. Mediation can help you attain some self-control. You get to eat the amount of food that your body requires.

Eating the recommended portion of food

Eating right can mean taking the amount of food that one needs. You find that certain chronic eating disorders prevent us from eating as we should. An individual with bulimia tends to consume more food than the required portion. There are various factors that can cause an individual to do so. For instance, they might be struggling with low self-esteem due to how they look. Some petite individuals wish they were a little bit bigger. As a result of their esteem issues, they end up consuming more than the required amount of food. There is a certain belief within them that if they eat a lot, they will get to the size they want. Sadly, that is not always the case. At times their body experiences no change, which can cause an individual to be frustrated. The same applies to eat less than the required amount of food. Skipping some meals is not good. You end up causing more harm to your body when you should be taking proper care of it. The best thing to do is to ensure that you take the recommended amount. This ensures that you stay healthy and fit. With the aid of mediation, you can maintain focus.

Consuming plant-based meals

Everyone should turn to eat vegetables. Plant-based meals contain nutrients that are helpful to our bodies. Some of the minerals present to ensure that our bodies are functioning as they should and normal body processes are being conducted well. The nutrients are effective in ensuring that we maintain good health by providing minerals that prevent certain diseases. Some of these minerals help in boosting the various metabolic processes occurring in our bodies. In case you have not been consuming plant-based meals, you have been missing a lot. Plant-based meals are also effective in weight loss. They ensure that we take only the right food portion that is helpful to our bodies. When most people want to start a weight loss journey, the immediate solution is talking plant-based meals. They have proven to be beneficial in that journey and process. In the past, people used to live long and were healthy because of consuming such diets. At this time, people would eat what they planted or what they hunted. They ate right and led a healthy life. One needs some discipline for them to eat plant-based meals.

Eat lightly cooked food

When we overcook meals, they do not have nutritious benefits to our bodies. You find that all the nutrients that were present are lost in the process. As you consume that food, it is not helpful to your body. Foods are beneficial when raw or when lightly cooked. Not everyone might manage to eat the foods when they are in this state. One needs some certain level of discipline for them to lightly cook their food and consume it in that state. At times you find that it is easier to consume food when fully cooked, especially with the taste that comes with it. You want to eat something sweet and something that you can easily chew. The problem with such desires is that the food will not help you in any way. At times you are torn between enjoying your meal or eating right. The two are difficult choices to choose from, and you may find yourself opting to enjoy your meal. Eating healthy can be fun, only if you tune your mind into it. Meditation will help you maintain focus, and you will easily accomplish the goals that you have set.

Reduce your sugar intake

Sugars are sweet and enticing. They make you want to eat more, and you simply cannot have enough of them. At times you crave to eat something that is sweet to your taste buds. The problem is the effect that these sugars have on your body. You find that when you consume them in excess, they cannot be utilized by the body. Instead of being converted into energy, they are converted into fats. When this happens, it can result in further complications to your body. We have some diseases such as diabetes that result from consuming excessive sugars. We also have some challenges, such as tooth problems that result from consuming sugars. At times they can be addictive, and all we wish to do is to take more of them. However, with the right discipline, we can regulate our sugar consumption. You can decide that you will be taking only a certain amount of sugars in a day. Meditation allows you to be focused on what you do. In this case, your focus is on regulating the number of sugars that you take. With this, you get to consume that which is necessary. In the end, it ensures that you have good health and that your body is in the right shape.

Avoid overeating

Overeating is a bad eating habit that everyone should avoid. In the process of overeating, one gets to add extra weight, and it has some harmful effects on their body. Mindful eating is essential in ensuring that we maintain good health. An individual's ability to focus can help them know when they are full. Different foods have different food components. There are some foods that will make you feel full at a fast rate than others will. You can analyze how your body feels after eating certain types of foods and know the effect of each food. This analysis helps you determine the portion that you should consume depending on the type of food involved. As a result, you make better and more informed decisions in terms of what you consume and watch the quantity that you take. To effectively follow this, one requires self-control that ensures they stick to the plan. This may appear like a challenging thing to accomplish, but it is possible with the help of meditation. You only need to tune your mind into consuming that which is necessary.

Chapter 11: Eating Mindlessly

We eat mindlessly. The principal explanation behind our awkwardness with nourishment and eating is that we have overlooked how to be available as we eat. Careful eating is the act of developing a receptive familiarity with how the nourishment we eat influences one's body, sentiments, brain, and all that is around us. The training improves our comprehension of what to eat, how to eat, the amount to eat, and why we eat what we eat. When eating carefully, we are completely present and relish each chomp connecting every one of our faculties to really value the nourishment. Past simple tastes, we see the appearance, sounds, scents, and surfaces of our nourishment, just as our mind's reaction to these perceptions.

The precepts of care apply to careful eating too; however, the idea of careful eating goes past the person. It likewise incorporates how what you eat influences the world. When we eat with this comprehension and understanding, appreciation and empathy will emerge inside us. Accordingly, careful eating is fundamental to guarantee nourishment supportability for who and what is to come, as we are persuaded to pick nourishments that are useful for our wellbeing, yet in addition useful for our planet.

It is outstanding that most get-healthy plans do not work in the long haul. Around 85% of individuals with heftiness who shed pounds come back to or surpass their underlying load inside a couple of years. Binge eating, passionate eating, outside seating, and eating because of nourishment longings have been connected to weight put on and weight recovers after effective weight reduction. Interminable presentation to stress may likewise assume an enormous job in gorging and heftiness. By changing the manner in which you consider nourishment, the negative sentiments that might be related to eating are supplanted with mindfulness, improved poise, and positive feelings. At the point when undesirable eating practices are tended to, your odds of long-haul weight reduction achievement are expanded.

Steps to Mindful Eating

1. Watch your shopping list

Do shopping mindfully, purchasing sound nourishments that are reasonably delivered and bundled is a significant piece of the training. One thing you will probably find about careful eating is that entire nourishments are more dynamic and heavenly than you may have given them acknowledgment for.

2. Figure out how to Eat Slower

Eating gradually does not need to mean taking it to limits. All things considered, it is a smart thought to remind yourself, and your family, that eating is not a race. Setting aside the effort to relish and make the most of your nourishment is perhaps the most advantageous thing you can do. You are bound to see when you are full, you'll bite your nourishment more and consequently digest it all the more effectively, and you'll likely end up seeing flavors you may some way or another have missed.

3. Eat when Necessary

It might take some training, however, locate that sweet spot between being eager and being ravenous to the point that you need to breathe in a dinner. Additionally, tune in to your body and get familiar with the distinction between being physically eager and sincerely ravenous. On the off chance that you skip dinners, you might be so anxious to get anything in your stomach that your first need is filling the void as opposed to making the most of your nourishment.

4. Enjoy your Senses

The vast majority partner eating with simply taste; and many eat so carelessly that even the taste buds get quick work. Be that as it may, eating is a blessing to a greater number of faculties than simply taste. When you are cooking, serving, and eating your nourishment, be mindful of shading, surface, fragrance, and even the sounds various nourishments make as you set them up. As you bite your nourishment, take a stab at distinguishing every one of the fixings, particularly seasonings. Eat with your fingers to give your feeling of touch some good times. By drawing in various faculties, the entire experience turns out to be significantly more completely fulfilling.

5. Keep off Distractions

Our day by day lives are brimming with interruptions, and it is normal for families to eat with the TV booming or one relative or another tinkering with their iPhone. Think about making family supper time, which should, obviously, be eaten together, a hardware-free zone. This does not mean eating alone peacefully; careful eating can be a great mutual encounter. It just means you do not eat before the TV, while driving, on the PC, on your telephone, and so on. Eating before the TV is for all intents and purposes the national hobby, however, simply consider how effectively it empowers careless eating.

6. Stop when you are Full

The issue with astounding nourishment is that by its very nature, it tends to be difficult to quit eating. Eating gradually will enable you to feel full before eating excessively, but on the other hand, it is imperative to be mindful of segment size and tune in to your body for when it starts disclosing to you it has had enough. Gorging may feel great at the time; however, it is awkward a short time later and is commonly not beneficial for the body. With a little practice, you can locate the without flaw spot between eating enough, however not all that much.

Careful eating does not need to be an activity in super-human focus, but instead a straightforward promise to acknowledging, regarding and, most importantly, getting a charge out of the nourishment you eat each day. It very well may be drilled with serving of mixed greens or frozen yogurt, doughnuts or tofu, and you can present it at home or at work. While the center turns out to be the means by which you eat, not what you eat, you may discover your thoughts of what you need to eat moving significantly for the better as well.

Meditating to Heal your Relationship with Food

The capacity to hold a wide scope of various feelings for the duration of the day is a test for a considerable lot of us. We simply need to feel upbeat, yet the test is to locate that mystical parity of all that we experience, decipher and do. The most regular history of past weight reduction endeavors is ceaseless confinements, which requires self-discipline and force. This perspective has a negative turn and does not draw out the best of us.

Meditation is a very accommodating device to mend enthusiastic eating. Meditation enables you to interface with your body. When you are in a condition of quiet and stillness, your state draws out the outer commotion of the world. Without these interruptions, it ends up simpler for you to drop into your body, construct, and support that association. When you have a solid association with your body, you are ready to accomplish things like unravel between physical yearning prompts versus enthusiastic appetite signals and perceive how to utilize nourishment for wellbeing and craving.

Stillness and predictable introduction to it enables you to construct your well of inward harmony and guidance. You will start to comprehend that you can exist outside of nourishment, weight, and everything in the middle. The more you reflect, the simpler you will discover it to drop into your body and associate with your higher self. You will be less inclined to go to binge eating as an approach to adapt to pressure and torment.

Meditation enables you to sharpen and use your breath. Breath resembles an inherent unwinding framework that you approach each moment of consistently. Breathing is the fastest method to accomplish a state change, which is the thing that your body is looking for when you voraciously consume food. Reflecting will condition you to depend on your breathing more on and then some, which means you will go after the shoddy nourishment less and less.

Make this a normal practice; ensure you do it consistently first and foremost. Since at that point, the requirement for nourishment to fill this hole of the void will not be as large as you discover delight from other progressively self-engaging sources. Mindfulness will develop and you will not just begin investigating yourself and your very own inward discussion, you will likewise expand your capacity to deal with the external mess. Obviously, it accepts practice likewise with each new routine, but it can likewise mend your association with nourishment.

Chapter 12: Consider Incorporating Working Out to Your Routine

The Rules of Working Out

That said, when you get going on a new exercise regimen, there are a few things you can keep in mind. These will help you get started and make sure you get the right kind of workout to suit your needs.

Firstly, the type of exercise you select will make a huge difference. To target your whole body, you need to be able to pick out a wide range of workouts. Cardio is the first form and you should spend three to four days a week getting some of this into your routine as it increases your heart rate and makes sure your heart gets some of the treatment it needs. Plus, the weight loss is really great because you can burn a lot of calories in the process.

That doesn't mean certain forms of workouts aren't important. Weight lifting can also be done a couple of days a week because it also strengthens those muscles. Your metabolism will burn much faster during the day while doing normal activities, when the muscles are toned up. So, while you may not burn as many calories as you do with cardio during the actual workout part, weight lifting can be amazing for the metabolism benefits.

And on stretching you can't forget. Take some time off your days, and do some stretching, like yoga or some other technique. This can help give the muscles a good time to relax after having worked so hard during the week, make them stronger and leaner and prevent injury.

Now, when it comes to how long you're supposed to work out, that will vary. When you want to lose weight, it's recommended you work out at least three days a week for 45 to 60 minutes. However, some people prefer to work out at whatever minutes for five or six days, so it's easier to fit into their schedule. When you are just beginning your fitness routine and it's been a while since you've worked out, beginning slowly would be better. Ten minutes is better than nothing and from there, you can build up. Never say you don't have time to work out; you can fit three or four ten-minute sessions into the day, and you've completed a full workout once you've done it.

Make sure the workouts you select have a lot of variety. Mix the stretching, cardio, and weight-lifting days together. Test out a host of different things, including some you've never done before. Mixing it up helps to focus on various muscle groups that help with weight loss and can make your workout easier to enjoy.

What if I don't have time to work out?

Some people worry they wouldn't have time to work out. They imagine spending hours at the gym to get the extra exercise you need to really see the results you like. Yet you don't need to waste all this time in the gym with Successful weight loss program. You just need to work out a few days a week, and then find other ways to fit into your routine a little bit of exercise. Some of the easy ways you can add to your routine in more movement include: Get up every hour, rather than sitting at your desk all day long and never moving, consider getting up every hour for at least two to five minutes. Walk around the room, do some jumping jacks and run around just a bit. For five minutes of an eight-hour day every hour, you'll end up for forty-five minutes of exercise. You too should bring this around. Do some sit-ups and pushups during commercial breaks during your favorite show and you will get an additional fifteen to twenty minutes each hour.

Park further away, if you need to take your vehicle, make sure you park far from the entrance. It might be just a few extra measures, but you do it a few times a day, and it really adds up.

Working out during your lunch break can be one of the best choices you can make. You can spend your lunch break just twenty minutes, and then enjoy a nutritious meal for the rest. This won't take too much of your time, so it can be a nice way to stroll around the office or work in the local gym without adjusting too much your schedule.

Take the stairs—if you're working in an office just below the first floor, try going up the stairs instead of the elevator. If the office is too far up to walk, start with a few flights and then take the rest of the way up the elevator. With time, you'll be able to increase your endurance and go up more flights of stairs.

Learn chair exercises, if you can't get up from your chair at work too often, learn a few basic exercises that will help you to work out your body without moving too often.

Add moves to chores—just cleaning the house can make you all sweaty. Make the movement intentional and add some things to it, and you're sure you'll get the additional exercise you want while making the house look fine.

Play at the park, take your kids to the park (walk there if you can) and then play at the park. Using the monkey bars, ride them, go down the slides and more. You'll be shocked to see how much of a workout this will end up for you.

There's still time to add more exercise to your day; for that to happen, you just need to be a little creative. If you get up more often from your chair or sneak a few times during the day in the workouts, you're sure to get the results you want.

The Benefits of Working Out

There are plenty of perks you'll reap when it comes to working out. You'll see a huge difference in the way your body behaves and responds, you'll be able to lower your stress levels and your attitude will begin to feel better in no time. Only ten minutes a day will make a major difference in the overall way you feel. Some of the great benefits you'll be able to see when you start working out include:

Better mood—it's time to have a workout on those days when you're just mad at everyone and grumpy... Even if you feel down and down, it's time to get out there and enjoy a good workout. Ten to fifteen minutes is all you need to make your mood feel better, and if you can work out for longer, you'll find that your body feels so much happier and satisfied when it's over.

Clearer mind—there's just something to figure out that will clean the mind out and make you feel so much better. When you feel foggy or you simply can't get any more work done for the day, and its only lunchtime, think about going out there and going into a good workout.

Healthier heart—your heart still wants some exercise. At least a few times a day, you want to use cardio to help the heart get up there and really get stronger. Also, if you have to start slowly, you will find in the beginning that working your heart with some good workouts like walking, running, swimming and cycling will help you get that heart in shape.

Faster weight loss—you eat calories while you work out. So, the more calories you eat up, the faster the weight loss becomes. Your metabolism should be quicker, and it can eat up all the excess fat the remains in the body, so you'll be able to see some of those weight loss results quicker than ever before.

Toned muscles—sitting on the couch doesn't help your muscles be safe and strong. Instead, it makes them frail and fragile and waste away. Neither do you just have to focus on weight lifting; stretching and cardio also have those muscles up and going, and you can see more strength in your body. Besides, these toned muscles will help speed up the metabolism, which is good whether or not you choose to lose weight.

Leaves you want more—beginning on an exercise plan may seem difficult at the beginning, and you may want to go out and do something else, you will learn to love it. If you can only keep up with the job for some time, you can see some amazing results in the process. You'll start looking forward to the workout, for instance, to see how many results you can achieve. If you're someone who gets bored with the workout, just have a plan every few months or so to change it and you're going to be perfect.

Although many people hate working out and putting all the time into it, there is actually a lot of good that can come from daily exercise. Give it a chance together with the other parts of your Successful weight loss program plan to see how much the outcomes will improve.

Chapter 13: Banning Food

The entire approach of intuitive eating revolves around listening to the body and keeping a finger on its pulse. If you are unable to follow the signals your body is giving out properly, then you are going to face problems in implementing this lifestyle. Any dietician that you go to initially or talk about with on the subject of intuitive eating will tell you that it's based on recognizing hunger and satisfying the needs accordingly. Earlier on, you read how there are different kinds of desire, and what you feel at times is not always what it seems like. Most of us are only familiar with physical hunger and spend our lives believing that it's the only type that exists.

The healthy living approach of intuitive eating has informed every one of us that this is not the case. Your body experiences varying forms of hunger, and they do not always have to be satisfied with the consumption of food. One of the first core principles of this philosophy teaches people to honor their hunger. This is about being aware of the biological urge which asks you to eat and then stop when you no longer feel empty. People say that at times, this can get confusing as, during the initial stages, one is still trying to train their body and mind. If you think about it, exploring where and what kind of hunger may not be as difficult as one would assume.

There are no technicalities or complications which you have to unravel. Just consider these few points:

• When you feel hungry, wherein your body can handle the physical sensation? Are your stomach wrenching and gnawing? If not, does your throat itch for something? Do you feel sluggish and tired? Sometimes, you might not experience any such thing but instead, start feeling weak and experiencing a headache. If this happens out of nowhere, it's a sign that your body needs to be replenished with nutrients.

• Does hunger affect your mood or concentration? Do you find yourself thinking of food in the middle of work or a conversation? Those who have answered yes to both these questions, well, there you have it. When you feel hungry, your mood changes for the worse, your ability to concentrate on any task hinders, and if your thoughts are going out to meals and snacks, then that is quite obvious.

• Are there any changes in your hunger when you travel, stressed, or functioning on low sleep? To determine those, you need to closely monitor your body and try to remedy the source of the change because a disturbance in the eating pattern may be emotional hunger rather than physical.

An integral aspect here which people should be mindful of is that everyone experiences or feels hunger differently, and what one person goes through does not apply to the other. Just remember that intuitive eating has no wrong answers, and it's a practice that brings about gradual progress, so if you do not get it instantly, there is nothing wrong with that because no one ever does.

Moving on to the other hunger, which we talked about that is emotional and does not require any satisfaction, which comes from food. There are four types of desire that people generally experience; real, which you should immediately respond to according to the intuitive eating philosophy, and then emotional, practical, and taste. In the beginning, you found out what physical and emotional hunger was about and how to successfully deal with each of them. Physical hunger is perhaps the most important one here as it's your body reaching out to you and sending cues. This is also something that a lot of people fail to pay adequate attention to. You see, the diet mentality and culture has led to many treating their necessary hunger as an enemy. They consider it as a challenge which has to be overcome because otherwise, it would result in shame and guilt. Well, how can something so essential and necessary for your survival be wrong for you? Hence, when your body begins to communicate with you, learn to listen.

Chapter 14: Tips for Great and Healthy Living

The ideal approach to accomplish better wellbeing is to change your way of life. It's tied in with causing a change from the nourishments you to eat to the exercises you do in your regular day to day existence. You can begin by staying away from lousy nourishments, slick, and handled food sources, since they will include more pounds into your body just as start setting aside some effort to work out.

This will empower you to have a better capacity to burn calories, which will help consume more fats just as get your body fit as a fiddle. This is only something you can do in remaining sound. To get more direction, simply read on as right now, we share with you tips on how you can begin your way towards a more useful life and you! Appreciate!

1. Sleep for at any rate of 8 hours every night.

Having enough rest part of the most significant activities to improve and keep up your wellbeing. It can make you increasingly vigorous the following day, besides the way that it can likewise forestall binge eating. All the more significantly, it is additionally perhaps the ideal approaches to prevent diseases, since it toughens your insusceptible framework.

2. Wash your hands as often as possible.

Washing your hands for the same number of times as you can for the entire day is perhaps the most ideal approach to forestall diseases. It ought to be finished with running water and a decent antibacterial cleanser. What's more, washing ought to be accomplished for in any event 20 seconds, to guarantee that it is liberated from any malady disease germs.

3. Never skip breakfast.

If your objectives are to get more benefits and to abstain from putting on an excessive amount of weight, at that point, skipping breakfast ought to be the keep going thing on your mind. Breakfast is the essential meal of the day. The feed can prop you up all consistently. If you skip it, odds are, you will put on weight because of binge eating and limited capacity to burn calories.

4. Drink, at any rate, eight glasses of water every day.

Water can help your body in flushing out poisons. Besides that, it can likewise guarantee that you are appropriately hydrated. Besides, drinking water can also help in stifling your hunger, which results in a fitter you. In this manner, make sure that you drink at any rate eight glasses of water each day to keep up your wellbeing.

5. Limit espresso consumption.

Espresso can now and again influence the nature of your absorption, which is the reason it ought not to be drilled all the time. A great many people drink various cups of espresso every day. To get more benefits, it is ideal if you chop it down to only one container for each day, or just to make drinking espresso a trivial thing.

6. Purchase a littler plate to either chop down your weight or to look after it.

Decreasing the measure of nourishments that you eat in every meal can have an emotional impact, with regards to keeping up or shedding pounds. Something you can accomplish for it is to buy a little plate, which is for your utilization as it were. With a bit of dish, you can fool yourself into eating littler segments, which would give you bunches of medical advantages over the long haul.

7. Try not to eat whatever isn't on your plate.

To acquire control on the measure of nourishments that you eat every day, it is ideal to abstain from eating nourishment that isn't on your plate. There are loads of occasions when you might need to get a bunch of peanuts out of the holder or take a sample of soup out of the bowl with a spoon. If you keep on doing this, at that point, you include more calories into your body without knowing it.

8. Eat-in a more slow way.

Eating quick is probably the ideal way if you need to put on more weight. Like this, you are doing something contrary to that can result in losing an abundance of pounds of weight. In this way, the time has come to make the most of your meals more by eating more slowly. At the point when you eat more slowly, you can stifle your craving, and it can likewise cause you to feel full, regardless of whether you have not expended a lot of nourishments yet after a specific timeframe.

9. Be sound emotionally.

As opposed to what a few people may accept, your feelings likewise assume an incredible job with regards to your wellbeing. In this manner, it is ideal if you can oversee it. As such, attempt to forestall blowing up, and consistently attempt to have an uplifting viewpoint of life. At the point when you do this, you can get more settled in most testing circumstances.

10. Think positive.

A few people may not trust it, yet your mind can influence your wellbeing in specific manners. For instance, if you generally imagine that you are becoming ill, at that point, it will build your odds of getting influenced by an ailment. Then again, if you believe that you are stable, at that point, you become increasingly dynamic, and it would likewise support your insusceptible framework.

11. Dodge popular fashion diets.

Most craze diets are diet programs, which are intended to cause individuals to get more fit quickly. By and large, these projects can include causing the individual to experience starvation, which can result in a quicker rate in getting more fit. In any case, because of the way that it has been accomplished, you can restore the weight in merely an issue of weeks, and you may even get heavier than when you previously began with it.

12. A brisk stroll for 3 to multiple times every week.

Energetic strolling is a movement that you can appreciate with your loved ones. It can help in boosting your digestion, which can result in weight loss. Besides that, it can likewise take care of business, your hips, bottom, just as your legs. Intend to energetic stroll for at any rate 20 minutes in 3 to 4 times each week, to pick up the advantages from it.

13. Exploit practice recordings.

If you are the sort of individual who wouldn't like to invest energy in driving, to find a right pace rec center, at that point, remind yourself that there are practice recordings that you can exploit. These recordings can be played at the solaces of your home whenever you need them. You should simply follow the schedules appeared in it and appreciate them.

14. Play with your children all the more frequently

Children are so lively, and we regularly wonder why. Be that as it may, if you play with them, you can help your vitality level too. This can result in a higher metabolic rate. In this manner, it can assist you with consuming more fats and calories, besides the way that doing it all the more frequently can likewise give you an approach to bond with them more.

15. Drink a glass of water when you wake up.

Drinking a glass of water after awakening offers a ton of medical advantages. For one, it gets your framework working, which can support up your vitality level. What's more, it can likewise help in purging your assemblage of poisons that have been aggregated for a long while.

16. Sharing is something that you ought not to do in ensuring your wellbeing.

With regards to your wellbeing, sharing ought not to be finished. This relates to the sharing of your things to different people, for example, hankies, toothbrushes, nail cutters, and such. The facts demonstrate that sharing is acceptable. However, this ought not to be watched about your own things.

17. Mind your pets.

A few people don't know that there are sure ailments, which can be transmitted from creatures to people. Along these lines, if you have pets, at that point, ensure that they are given their suggested inoculations. What's more, you ought to likewise make sure that they are appropriately prepped, with the goal that they are liberated from ticks and bugs that may also convey germs.

18. Try not to confound ache to hunger.

There are times when we open up our coolers to get a bite, in any event, when our body is aching for water. This is because we tend to decipher thirst as appetite. Consequently, if you want to eat in any event, when you have quite recently had your meal, at that point, attempt to drink a glass of water. By and large, you will feel fulfilled as a result of it, particularly since you were dehydrated in any case.

19. Maintain a strategic distance from prepared nourishments as much as you can.

Handled nourishments like franks, burgers, French fries, and such don't contain enough supplements to furnish your body with what it needs. Besides that, they are likewise topped off with a ton of artificial flavorings, which can make your body amass bunches of poisons. Therefore, it is ideal for evading them for as much as you can. Staying away from them can help forestall maladies, besides the way that it would likewise help in making you more beneficial.

20. Eat nourishments that are high in fiber content.

If one of your wellbeing objectives is to shed a couple of pounds, at that point load up on fiber, fiber draws out the absorption procedure, which implies that it can cause you to feel full more. At the point when that occurs, you usually are stifling your hunger. Besides that, fiber can likewise help in freeing your assortment of waste.

21. Cut down your utilization of carbonated sodas.

Carbonated sodas are stacked with a great deal of sugar, which can make you put on weight, and it can even build your odds of getting diabetic. A few people who are partial to drinking such refreshments incline toward diet ones since they guarantee to contain lesser measures of sugar. Be that as it may, such beverages are stacked with aspartame, which can cause heaps of medical problems over the long haul.

22. Utilize the stairs rather than the lift.

At whatever point you report to your office, make it a propensity to utilize the stairs rather than the lift. This can offer an original route for you to consume more fats and calories. It is a type of activity, which can fortify your leg muscles, and it is a decent option in contrast to running or lively strolling.

23. Eat more organic products.

Organic products are stacked with natural nutrients and dampness to keep you feeling better. It is perhaps the ideal approach to forestall ailments and blockage. Most organic products additionally contain chemicals that help your body in engrossing the supplements offered by the nourishments that you eat.

Chapter 15: The Rapid Weight Loss: Good or Bad?

No nourishment is taboo when you pursue this arrangement, which doesn't make you purchase any prepackaged suppers.

Rapid Weight Loss appoints different nourishments Point esteem. Nutritious nourishments that top you off have less focuses than garbage with void calories. The eating plan factors sugar, fat, and protein into its focuses counts to direct you toward natural products, veggies, and lean protein and away from stuff that is high in sugar and immersed fat.

You'll have a Point focus on that is set up dependent on your body and objectives. For whatever length of time that you remain inside your everyday target, you can spend those Points anyway you'd like, even on liquor or treat, or spare them to utilize one more day.

However, more beneficial, lower-calorie nourishments cost less focuses. Furthermore, a few things presently have o points.

Level of Effort: Medium

Rapid Weight Loss is intended to make it simpler to change

your propensities long haul, and it's adaptable enough that you ought to have the option to adjust it to your life. You'll improve your eating and lifestyle designs a considerable lot of which you may have had for quite a long time and you'll make new ones.

How much exertion it takes relies upon the amount you'll need to change your propensities.

Cooking and shopping: Expect to figure out how to shop, cook solid nourishments, and eat out in manners that help your weight-loss objective without holding back on taste or expecting to purchase strange nourishments.

Bundled nourishments or dinners: Not required.

In-person gatherings: Optional.

Exercise: You'll get a customized action objective and access to the program's application that tracks Points. You get acknowledgment for the entirety of your action.

Does It Allow for Dietary Restrictions or Preferences?

Because you pick how you spend your Points, you can at present do Rapid Weight Loss if you're a veggie-lover, vegetarian, have different inclinations, or if you have to confine salt or fat.

What Else You Should Know

Cost: Rapid Weight Loss offers three plans: Online just, online with gatherings, or online with one-on-one training through telephone calls and messages. Check the Rapid Weight Loss site for the evaluation of "online just" and "online with gatherings" alternatives (you'll have to enter your ZIP code).

Costs and offers may differ.

Backing: Besides the discretionary in-person gatherings (presently called health workshops) and individual instructing, Rapid Weight Loss Program has an application, an online network, a magazine, and a site with plans, tips, examples of overcoming adversity, and that's only the tip of the iceberg.

Does It Work?

Rapid Weight Loss is one of the well-looked into weight loss programs accessible. What's more, indeed, it works.

Numerous studies have demonstrated that the arrangement can assist you with getting more fit and keep it off.

For example, an investigation from The American Journal of Medicine demonstrated that individuals making Rapid Weight Loss lost more weight than those attempting to drop beats without anyone else.

Rapid Weight Loss positioned first both for "Best Weight Loss Diet" and for "Best Commercial Diet Plan" in the 2018 rankings from U.S. News and World Report.

Generally speaking, it's a great, simple to-pursue program.

Is It Good for Certain Conditions?

Rapid Weight Loss is useful for anybody. In any case, its attention on nutritious, low-calorie nourishments makes it extraordinary for individuals with hypertension, elevated cholesterol, diabetes, and even coronary illness.

If you pick any premade dinners, check the names, as some might be high in sodium.

Please work with your primary care physician so they can check your advancement, as well. This is particularly significant for individuals with diabetes, as you may need to alter your medication as you get in shape.

If the idea of gauging your nourishment or checking calories makes your head turn, this is a perfect program because it takes every necessary step for you. The online instrument allocates a specific number an incentive to every nourishment, even eatery nourishments, to make it simple to remain on track.

If you don't have the foggiest idea about your way around the kitchen, the premade dinners and bites make it simple. They're a speedy and simple approach to control partition sizes and calories.

You don't need to drop any nourishment from your eating routine, yet you should constrain divide sizes to curtail calories.

The accentuation on foods grown from the ground implies the eating routine is high in fiber, which helps keep you full. Also, the program is easy to pursue, making it simpler to adhere to. You can likewise discover Rapid Weight Loss Program premade dinners at your neighborhood market.

A major favorable position of Rapid Weight Loss is their site. They offer exhaustive data on abstaining from excessive food intake, exercise, cooking, and wellness tips, just as online care groups.

Beset up to go through some cash to get the full advantages of the vigorous program. It tends to be somewhat expensive, yet it's well justified, despite all the trouble to harvest the wellbeing advantages of getting more fit and keeping it off.
Part Benefits

Dieters who join Rapid weight loss are known as "individuals."

Individuals can browse a few projects with differing levels of help.

An essential online program incorporates every minute of every day online visit support, just as applications and different instruments. Individuals can pay more for face to face bunch gatherings or one-on-one help from a Rapid weight loss individual mentor.

Individuals additionally get access to an online database of thousands of nourishments and plans, notwithstanding the following application for logging Points.

Also, Rapid weight loss supports physical action by relegating a wellness objective utilizing Points.

Every action can be signed into the Rapid weight loss application until the client arrives at their week after week FitPoint objective.

Exercises like moving, strolling and cleaning would all be able to be tallied towards your Point objective.

Rapid weight loss additionally gives wellness recordings and exercise schedules for their individuals.

Alongside diet and exercise directing, Rapid weight loss sells bundled nourishment like solidified suppers, cereal, chocolates and low-calorie dessert.

Outline

Rapid weight loss doles out guide esteems toward nourishments. Individuals must remain under their assigned day by day nourishment and drink focuses to meet their weight-misfortune objectives.

Would it be able to Help You Lose Weight?

Rapid weight loss utilizes a science-based way to deal with weight misfortune, accentuating the significance of part control, nourishment decisions and moderate, predictable weight misfortune.

Dissimilar to numerous craze diets that guarantee unreasonable outcomes over brief timeframes, Rapid weight loss discloses to individuals that they ought to hope to lose .5 to 2 pounds (.23 to .9 kg) every week.

The program features lifestyle modification and advice individuals on the best way to settle on better choices by utilizing the Points framework, which organizes sound nourishments.

Numerous studies have demonstrated that Rapid weight loss can help with weight misfortune.

Rapid weight loss gives a whole page of their site to scientific examinations supporting their program.

One study found that overweight individuals who were advised to get more fit by their PCPs lost twice as a lot of weight on the Rapid weight loss program than the individuals who got standard weight misfortune directing from essential care proficient.

Even though this investigation was subsidized by Rapid weight loss, information gathering, and examination were facilitated by a free research group.

Besides, an audit of 39 controlled examinations found that members following the Rapid weight loss program lost 2.6% more weight than members who got different sorts of guidance.

Another controlled investigation in more than 1,200 hefty grown-ups found that members who pursued the Rapid weight loss program for one year lost significantly more weight than the individuals who got self-improvement materials or brief weight-misfortune counsel.

Besides, members following Rapid weight loss for one year were increasingly fruitful at keeping up their weight misfortune for more than two years, contrasted with different gatherings.

Rapid weight loss is one of only a handful scarcely any weight-misfortune programs with demonstrated outcomes from randomized controlled preliminaries, which are considered the "best quality level" of therapeutic research.

Conclusion

Let's look back at our progress and then paying it forward to others. Continue eating better all day. You'll feel better, look better, achieve your goals, and have a better quality of life. Assuming you've read and understood all the content here, chances are that you've realized your habits and applying core solutions to overcoming obstacles while holding yourself accountable, you have Paid attention to yourself, your purpose, unique talents, and dreams. By automating your food and water, cutting out unhealthy sugar, alcohol and white carbs, adding protein, Greek yogurt or other probiotics, produce and healthy fats.

Choose to continue with the same eating habit all your life. Focus on a healthy weight; stay with silence. Visualize your step and take steps that are going to get you to where you want to be. If you destabilize procrastination, stress and comfort zone, you will go farther at a fast pace. Organize your kitchen and automate your food. Be a reader; Read positive affirmations aloud every day. Pursue your goals, including your fitness and health goals that will utilize your talents and passions and keep you on the healthy-fit journey. Rest on weekends and follow the process again.

Focus on your activities, journalize your progress, thoughts, and move on. Record your success, nature; they will guide you in thinking and solving stress, among other problems. You will make not only an impact on yourself but also the people around you. Make use of productivity apps on the internet to guide you through.

While writing your journal, consider how you've grown physically, mentally, spiritually, and emotionally or socially. Think about how one area has positively affected other areas. If some things haven't worked out for you, spend some time forgiving other people, forgiving yourself so you can move on. Giving makes living worthwhile.

Albert Einstein believed that a life shared with others is worthy. We have people out there who need you, remember not to hoard your successes. Share your success. Share your new-found recipes, your attitude, and your habits. Share what you have learned with others. In all your undertakings, know that you can't change other people but yourself, therefore, be mindful. Reflect on your changes and put yourself on the back today and every day. Be grateful and live your life as a champion.

Make it a reality on your mind, the fact that the journey to a healthy life and weight loss is long and has many challenges. Pieces of Stuff we consider more important in life require our full cooperation towards them. Just because you are facing problems in your Wight loss journey, it does not mean that you should stop, instead show and prove the whole world how good your ability to handle constant challenges is—training your brain to know that eating healthy food together with functional exercises can work miracles. Make it your choice and not something you are forced to do by a third party. Always tell yourself that weight loss is a long process and not an event. Take every day of your days to celebrate your achievements because these achievements are what piles up to a massive victory. Make a list of stuff you would like to change when you get healthy they may be Small size-clothes, being able to accumulate enough energy, participating in your most loved sports you have been admiring for a more extended period, feeling self-assured. Make these tips your number one source of empowerment; you will end up completing your 30 days even without noticing.

You have made it, or you are about to make it. The journey has been unbelievable. And by now, you must be having a story to tell. Concentrate on finishing strongly. Keep up the excellent eating design you have adopted. Remember, you are not working on temporary changes but long-term goals. Therefore, lifestyle changes should not be stopped when the weight is lost. Remind yourself always of essential habits that are easier to follow daily. They include trusting yourself and the process by acknowledging that the real change lies in your hands. Stop complacency, arise, and walk around for at least thirty minutes away. Your breakfast is the most important meal you deserve. Eat your breakfast like a queen. For each diet, you take, add a few proteins and natural fats. Let hunger not kill you, eat more, but just what is recommended, bring snacks and other meals 3 or 5 times a day. Have more veggies and fruits like 5-6 rounds in 24 hours. Almost 90% of Americans do not receive enough vegetables and fruits to their satisfaction. Remember, Apple will not make you grow fat. Substitute salt. You will be shocked by the sweet taste of food once you stop consuming salt. Regain your original feeling, you will differentiate natural flavorings from artificial flavors. Just brainstorm how those older adults managed to eat their food without salt or modern-day characters. Characters are not suitable for your health. Drink a lot of water in a day. Let water be your number one drink. Avoid soft drinks and other energy drinks, and they are slowly killing you. Drink a lot of water in the morning after getting out of your bed. Your body will be fresh from morning to evening. Have a journal and be realistic with it. Take charge of what you write and be responsible.